THE CANCER ATLAS

Second Edition

Ahmedin Jemal
Paolo Vineis
Freddie Bray
Lindsey Torre
David Forman

International Agency for Research on Cancer

World Health Organization

Published by the American Cancer Society, Inc.
250 Williams Street
Atlanta, Georgia 30303 USA
www.cancer.org

ISBN-10: 1-60443-228-4
ISBN-13: 978-1-60443-228-2

Printed in China
1 2 3 4 5   14 15 16 17 18

LIBRARY OF CONGRESS CATALOGING-IN-PUBLICATION DATA
The cancer atlas / Ahmedin Jemal [and four others]. — Second edition.
p. cm.
Includes bibliographical references.
ISBN 978-1-60443-228-2 (pbk.) — ISBN 1-60443-228-4 (pbk.)
1. Cancer--Atlases. 2. Cancer—Epidemiology.
I. Jemal, Ahmedin.
RC262.C274 2015
616.99'4--dc23
2014032148

Managing Editor: John M. Daniel
Design: Language Dept. (*www.languagedept.com*)
Contributing Editor: Kimberly D. Miller

SUGGESTED CITATION:
Jemal A, Vineis P, Bray F, Torre L, Forman D (Eds). *The Cancer Atlas*. Second Ed.
Atlanta, GA: American Cancer Society; 2014. Also available at: www.cancer.org/
canceratlas.

The Cancer Atlas can be found online at *www.cancer.org/canceratlas*.
The online version of the Atlas provides additional resources and information unique
to the online interactive edition.

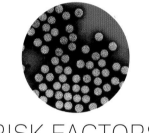
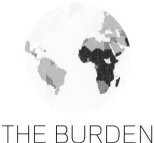

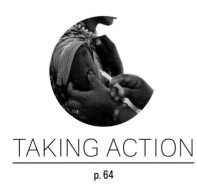

TAKING ACTION

*The findings and conclusions in this publication
are those of the authors and do not necessarily represent the official
position of the Centers for Disease Control and Prevention.

"One of the great cancer control challenges of the 21st century is to bring the benefits of effective interventions to as many people as possible, including in low- and middle-income countries."

—*Christopher Wild, Director, International Agency for Research on Cancer*

JOHN R. SEFFRIN

Chief Executive Officer,
American Cancer Society

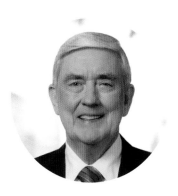

There has perhaps never been a more exciting time to be part of the fight against cancer. Never before have we faced such great challenge, or such great opportunity, in our work to combat this disease worldwide and to ultimately bring it under control.

In recent years, we have made marked progress against cancer in many countries. In the USA, for example, we have seen 20 successive years of declines in cancer mortality rates, which translates to a total of more than 1.3 million cancer deaths averted.

Yet as you will see in the pages of this *Atlas*, in far too many corners of the globe, cancer threatens lives and livelihoods as never before. Africa, for example, is poised to become the epicenter of the tobacco pandemic, which threatens to kill 1 billion this century, if left unchecked— many of those deaths from cancer. Other regions are threatened by this scourge as well. And across the map, low- and middle-income nations are struggling with how to effectively turn the tide against the rising threat of cancer and other chronic diseases, which is burdening ill-prepared health care systems and emerging economies alike.

If we are to bring cancer under control as a major public health problem, it will take all of us, working together, to do so. We must work across all sectors, and learn from and with one another, sharing the proven strategies and best buys we've developed while fighting this disease. The American Cancer Society is so pleased to participate in this second edition of *The Cancer Atlas* because it embodies this spirit of collaboration and the open exchange of information that must take place if we are to save more lives.

We at the Society believe this critical publication will be an essential and accessible resource for everyone involved in the cancer fight—from advocates and agencies to policymakers and patients, and everyone in between. This timely, evidence-based publication offers a wealth of compelling data to help combat cancer in communities and nations worldwide. Information is a powerful tool in the hands of passionate, dedicated individuals, and this book provides an unparalleled resource to arm and inform everyone committed to this fight.

This edition of *The Cancer Atlas* is unique because it brings together expert opinions from around the globe, with more than 40 contributing authors and peer reviewers. Just as it is designed as a resource for diverse groups, so too do the contributing experts come from diverse backgrounds, ranging from centers of academia to government institutions and nongovernmental organizations. It is also unique in its accessibility, as the *Atlas* will be available for the first time in an interactive and free online edition.

The American Cancer Society is committed to working relentlessly to save more lives from cancer both at home and worldwide, and to one day finishing this fight for good. We believe this second edition of *The Cancer Atlas* will be a valuable tool that helps us all work collectively toward this laudable— and achievable— goal. As you peruse the pages that follow, I am sure you will agree.

> **"**
>
> ***[The Cancer Atlas]* brings together expert opinions from around the globe, with more than 40 contributing authors and peer reviewers. Just as it is designed as a resource for diverse groups, so too do the contributing experts come from diverse backgrounds.**

CARY ADAMS

Chief Executive Officer, Union for International Cancer Control

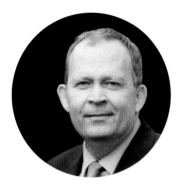

In September 2011 at the United Nations in New York, all countries committed to a Political Declaration on non-communicable diseases (NCDs), which many commentators suggested put cancer on the global health agenda for the very first time. It was only the second United Nations high-level meeting on a health issue —the previous one being on HIV/AIDS in 2001— and expectations were high that this significant event would be a turning point in the way cancer and the other NCDs would be addressed in future years in all countries.

Since then, the World Health Organization has marshalled member states through a three-year process that has resulted in agreement to a global goal to reduce premature deaths from cancer and the other NCDs by 25% by 2025, a refreshed Global Action Plan on NCDs, and a large number of targets and indicators to be adopted by countries to measure their progress in delivering a dramatic change in the morbidity and mortality of cancer around the globe. A combination of effective advocacy, dynamic leadership from some countries and the infusion of great evidence and data at the appropriate junctures has placed cancer on the global health map for the very first time.

The Union for International Cancer Control believes that we have sufficient knowledge on cancer prevention, early detection, and treatment services for cure and improving quality of life to achieve the goals set out by the United Nations, which we have now embedded in a refreshed World Cancer Declaration launched in Cape Town in November 2013. What we need is the engagement of governments and national cancer leaders around the world to put that knowledge into practice—wholeheartedly addressing cancer risk factors like tobacco use, implementing population-based vaccination and screening programs, reducing the myths, misconceptions and stigma so often associated with cancer through comprehensive education programs, and improving the way in which primary care informs and engages patients to encourage the early presentation of the disease. These steps do not need breakthrough science to be effective. They demand the application of known interventions which are effective in all situations, as well as the transfer of knowledge so the challenge of cancer becomes manageable in the minds of the many.

The Cancer Atlas is an important tool in our ambition to engage with communities around the world to convey the facts about a disease that is misunderstood by many who we hope will commit to address the disease in their country. The *Atlas* informs in a very clear and concise way the challenges faced in dealing with cancer around the world. It is a valuable addition to the toolkit of the advocate, the library of the oncologist, the knowledge of the patient, the resource base of the journalist, the database of government officials and scientists. The Union for International Cancer Control and its membership in more than 150 countries will ensure that the *Atlas* is available to all those committed to improve national cancer control planning. I am delighted that working with our partners the American Cancer Society and the International Agency for Research on Cancer, we have been able bring together such an impressive publication to inform the world.

> "
> **The Cancer Atlas is an important tool in our ambition to engage with communities around the world to convey the facts about a disease that is misunderstood by many who we hope will commit to address the disease in their country.**

CHRISTOPHER WILD

Director, International Agency for Research on Cancer

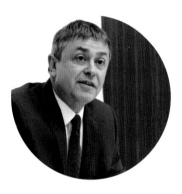

We cannot treat our way out of the cancer problem. In even the wealthiest countries, the social and economic burden of cancer exacts a cost that cannot be met through improvements in therapy alone, however much targeted and refined to exploit the underlying molecular basis of the disease. Such necessary emphasis on clinical care must be complemented by public health measures, which include cancer prevention, early detection and diagnosis. The second edition of *The Cancer Atlas* serves as an outstanding reference both in content and form, providing a reliable foundation for action across the full spectrum of cancer control measures.

The first step to prevention is an understanding of the causes, and in this context *The Cancer Atlas* provides a valuable summary of major cancer risk factors, emphasizing the geographic variation in their prevalence. This theme of heterogeneity is continued in the descriptions of the regional variation in cancer burden. A clear picture of cancer incidence, mortality, survival and prevalence at regional and national levels is a vital platform for cancer control planning. Without such information there is a major risk of misplaced emphasis and wasted investment. *The Cancer Atlas* draws on the sources available, notably the International Agency for Research on Cancer's GLOBOCAN database, but also provides a reminder of how much progress is still required in establishing reliable population-based cancer registries in many low- and middle-income countries where data remain sparse. This paucity of data on occurrence also extends to include information on many of the risk factors. In this sense, this valuable publication can also be viewed as a call to greater action in these areas of surveillance.

The Cancer Atlas not only describes the problem but relates some of the available solutions, encompassing primary prevention, screening and early detection, treatment and palliative care. This comprehensive approach provides a balanced picture of what could be achieved already if the scientific evidence were to be translated into practice. Perhaps the most striking message from *The Cancer Atlas*, however, is not the variation in occurrence of risk factors and cancer patterns but the inequalities in access to the very interventions that can either prevent or effectively treat and manage the disease. This inequality is seen both between and within countries, and it is visible in respect to all aspects of cancer control and management. In relation to cancer, where you live affects your risk of developing the disease, how you live with the disease, and ultimately whether you survive the disease. One of the great cancer control challenges of the 21st century is to bring the benefits of effective interventions to as many people as possible, including in low- and middle-income countries.

Cancer is a barrier to sustainable human development. This important conclusion is now being recognized at international and national levels, not least because of the emphasis placed by the United Nations on non-communicable diseases (NCDs). This political recognition must be translated to changing priorities, particularly in relation to expenditure on development assistance for health, where donors to date have paid little attention to cancer and other NCDs. Here I am convinced *The Cancer Atlas* will provide its greatest value, in its superb presentation of reliable information in an accessible, useable format for decision-makers, advocates, patients and the general public. I am confident, therefore, that the collaboration between the American Cancer Society, the Union for International Cancer Control, and the International Agency for Research on Cancer on *The Cancer Atlas* can be an agent for change in cancer control on a global scale.

> ❝
>
> **The most striking message is not the variation in occurrence of risk factors and cancer patterns but the inequalities in access to the very interventions that can either prevent or effectively treat and manage**

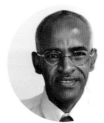

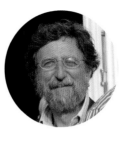

AHMEDIN JEMAL

Dr. Jemal is Vice President of the Surveillance & Health Services Research Program at the American Cancer Society. He also holds an appointment as adjunct Associate Professor of Epidemiology at the Rollins School of Public Health, Emory University.

Dr. Jemal's principal research interests include cancer disparities and the social determinants of health and health services and outcomes research, with a focus on major cancers and common risk factors. His main goal at the American Cancer Society has been to build a strong team of cancer surveillance and health services researchers to promote the application of evidence-based cancer prevention and control in the USA and worldwide. Dr. Jemal has published more than 150 articles in peer-reviewed journals.

PAOLO VINEIS

Dr. Vineis, Professor and Chair of Environmental Epidemiology at Imperial College, London, is a leading researcher in the field of molecular epidemiology. His latest research activities mainly focus on examining biomarkers of disease risk, complex exposures, and intermediate biomarkers from "omic" platforms (including metabolomics and epigenetics) in large epidemiological studies. He has more than 700 publications (many as leading author) in journals such as *Nature, Nature Genetics, Lancet,* and *Lancet Oncology*. He is a member of numerous international scientific and ethics committees.

Professor Vineis has extensive experience in leading international projects. He is coordinating the European Commission-funded Exposomics Project, and he is a Principal Investigator/Co-investigator of numerous international projects, such as the European Commission funded GENAIR, ECNIS2, Envirogenomarkers, Hypergenes, ESCAPE and Transphorm projects. In addition, he has attracted grants from the Leverhulme Trust, MRC, Cancer Research UK, HuGeF Foundation, and the US National Cancer Institute. He is the director of the Unit of Molecular and Genetic Epidemiology, HuGeF Foundation, Torino, Italy, and leads the Exposome and Health Programme of the MRC-PHE Centre for Environment and Health at Imperial College.

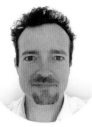

FREDDIE BRAY

Dr. Bray is Head of the Cancer Surveillance Section at the International Agency for Research on Cancer (IARC), in Lyon, France. He previously worked at the Cancer Registry of Norway and University of Oslo from 2005 to 2010 and again at IARC from 1998 to 2005. He has a PhD in Epidemiology from the London School of Hygiene and Tropical Medicine, and degrees in statistics from the University of Aberdeen and in medical statistics from the University of Leicester, United Kingdom. His areas of research revolve around the descriptive epidemiology of cancer, including the estimation of the global cancer burden, the analysis of time trends, and global predictions of the future scale and profile of cancer linked to human development transitions. He has close to 200 book chapters and articles in journals including *The Lancet, Lancet Oncology,* the *Journal of the National Cancer Institute,* and *Nature Reviews Cancer.*

In support of the overwhelming need for high quality cancer surveillance systems, Dr. Bray leads the Global Initiative for Cancer Registration (*http://gicr.iarc.fr*), an international multi-partner program designed to ensure a sustainable expansion of the coverage and quality of population-based cancer registries in low- and middle-income countries through tailored, localized support and advocacy to individual countries.

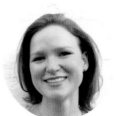

LINDSEY TORRE

Ms. Torre joined the Surveillance Research group at the American Cancer Society as an epidemiologist in 2012. She concentrates on global cancer surveillance. She is lead author of Global Cancer Facts & Figures, 3rd edition, which is slated for release in 2015, and also conducts and collaborates on research focused on global cancer control, with particular emphasis on risk factors and disparities.

Ms. Torre received a BS (2004) in International Political Economy from Georgetown University, and an MSPH (2012) in Global Epidemiology from the Rollins School of Public Health, Emory University. Prior to joining the American Cancer Society, she worked in implementation of HIV prevention and reproductive health programs internationally.

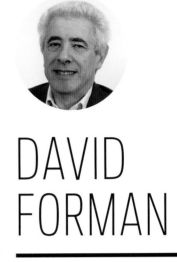

DAVID FORMAN

Dr. Forman was, until mid-2014, Head of the Cancer Information Section at the International Agency for Research on Cancer (IARC) in Lyon, France. This Section of IARC is responsible for providing information concerning worldwide cancer vital statistics and produces the definitive reference source "Cancer Incidence in Five Continents (CI5)". Part of this responsibility includes supporting cancer registries worldwide, especially in low- and medium-resource countries. The Section also maintains an active research program in the descriptive epidemiology of cancer. Prior to taking up his appointment at IARC in April 2010, Dr. Forman was, from 1994, Professor of Cancer Epidemiology at the University of Leeds, UK, and Director of the Northern and Yorkshire Cancer Registry. He was also Head of Analysis and Information for the UK National Cancer Intelligence Network. From 1982 to 1994, he was a Staff Scientist with the Imperial Cancer Research Fund Epidemiology Unit in Oxford, UK, working initially with Sir Richard Doll. Dr. Forman's PhD and postdoctoral research was in cancer biology.

Dr. Forman's research profile includes studies in the epidemiology of cancer, and he has also been involved in health services research in cancer and, in association with the Cochrane Collaboration, systematic reviews and meta-analyses in upper gastrointestinal disease. Much of his research has been focused on cancers of the gastrointestinal tract, and he has been particularly identified with studies examining the association between stomach cancer and *H. pylori* infection. He has over 250 publications in peer-reviewed journals and remains based at IARC as a Senior Visiting Fellow.

ACKNOWLEDGEMENTS

The editors of *The Cancer Atlas*, Second Edition would like to thank the American Cancer Society and the International Agency for Research on Cancer for their support of this edition.
We would also like to thank the Union for International Cancer Control for their generous support of the online version of this edition.

Many individuals have donated their time and expertise in the preparation of the Atlas. In particular, we would like to thank **Mathieu Laversanne** at the International Agency for Research on Cancer for supplying datasets and invaluable analytical support. For their individual contributions to the Atlas, we would like to thank **Rebecca Siegel, Jennifer Greenwald, Elizabeth Mendes, and Kerri Gober** at the American Cancer Society, and **Michel Coleman** at the London School of Hygiene and Tropical Medicine.

We would also like to express our deep appreciation for our authors and peer reviewers. Our peer reviewers include:

- **Rachel Ballard-Barbash,** National Cancer Institute (USA)
- **H. Bas Bueno-de-Mesquita,** National Institute of Public Health and the Environment (The Netherlands)
- **Eduardo Cazap,** Sociedad Latino Americana y del Caribe de Oncologia Medica
- **Graham Colditz,** Washington University Institute for Public Health and School of Medicine
- **Vera Luiza da Costa e Silva,** National Public Health School, Oswaldo Cruz Foundation
- **Paul Dickman,** Karolinska Institutet, Department of Medical Epidemiology and Biostatistics
- **Brenda Edwards,** National Cancer Institute (USA)
- **Tom Glynn,** American Cancer Society Cancer Action Network
- **Michael Hanlon,** University of Washington, Institute for Health Metrics and Evaluation
- **Joe Harford,** National Cancer Institute (USA)
- **Rolando Herrero Acosta,** International Agency for Research on Cancer
- **Mazda Jenab,** International Agency for Research on Cancer
- **Prabhat Jha,** St. Michael's Hospital and University of Toronto, Centre for Global Health Research
- **Tim Key,** University of Oxford, Cancer Epidemiology Unit
- **Jane Kim,** Harvard School of Public Health, Program in Health Decision Science
- **Martha Linet,** National Cancer Institute (USA)
- **Joannie Lortet-Tieulent,** American Cancer Society
- **Max Parkin,** University of Oxford
- **Neil Pearce,** London School of Hygiene and Tropical Medicine
- **Petra Peeters,** Imperial College London, School of Public Health
- **Michael Peake,** National Cancer Intelligence Network (UK)
- **Paola Pisani,** University of Torino
- **M.R. Rajagopal,** Pain and Palliative Care Clinic, Medical College, Calicut
- **Jonathan Samet,** University of Southern California, Institute for Global Health
- **Robert Smith,** American Cancer Society
- **Lisa Stevens,** National Cancer Institute (USA)
- **Bernard Stewart,** Cancer Control Program, South Eastern Sydney Public Health Unit
- **Diane Summers,** GAVI Alliance Secretariat
- **Catherine Thomson,** Information Services Division Scotland
- **Edward Trimble,** National Cancer Institute (USA)
- **Margaret Tucker,** National Cancer Institute (USA)
- **Walter Willett,** Harvard School of Public Health
- **Martin Wiseman,** World Cancer Research Fund International

A number of individuals and organizations provided additional expertise on specific chapters:

- **Recinda Sherman,** North American Association of Central Cancer Registries
- **Jonathan Lieberman,** McCabe Centre, Melbourne
- **Peter Campbell** and **Alpa Patel,** American Cancer Society
- **Leanne Riley** and **Melanie Cowan,** World Health Organization
- **Dana Schneider,** Centers for Disease Control and Prevention (USA)

Finally, for their diverse talents and design expertise, we would like to thank the team at Language Dept.: **Jenn Cash, Tanya Quick, Lizania Cruz, Leah Koransky, Angela Choi,** and **Niquita Taliaferro**.

This 2nd edition of *The Cancer Atlas* represents a comprehensive global overview of information about the burden of cancer, associated risk factors, methods of prevention and measures of control. *The Atlas* maintains the structure of the first edition, published in 2006, with chapters grouped into three sections: risk factors, the burden, and taking action.

RISK FACTORS

The first section highlights the magnitude of regional and international variations in many of the major risk factors for cancer, ① including tobacco use, ② infections, unhealthy diet, and ultraviolet radiation. Tobacco use continues to be the predominant established cause of cancer in most high-income countries, while infections play a major role in many sub-Saharan African and Asian countries. ③ The importance of obesity as a major risk factor for cancer is growing in most parts of the world, now including low- and middle-income countries.

Some of the Major Cancer Risk Factors

Environmental Pollutants

Tobacco

Diet and Obesity

Occupational Carcionagens

Infections

Reproductive Habits

④
World Human Development Index

②
Infections

①

Tobacco Use

③
Unhealthy Diets

THE BURDEN

④ The section on the cancer burden has been substantially expanded since the first edition, with dedicated chapters for all major world regions, and these chapters reveal the striking geographic diversity in the pattern of different cancers. Also described are the burden according to the Human Development Index, and the burden in terms of years of life lost (YLL), a measure that gives more weight to deaths occurring at younger ages.

TAKING ACTION

⑤ The section on taking action describes the major types of intervention across the cancer continuum, from prevention of risk factors to early detection, treatment and palliative care, as well as the disparities in application of these interventions across the world. It also ⑥ provides descriptions of organizations working in cancer control and recent policies and legislation to address cancer and other non-communicable diseases.

The Cancer Atlas is intended to provide basic information on the global burden of cancer in user-friendly and accessible form for cancer control advocates, government and private public health agencies and policy makers as well as patients, survivors and the general public in order to promote cancer prevention and control worldwide.

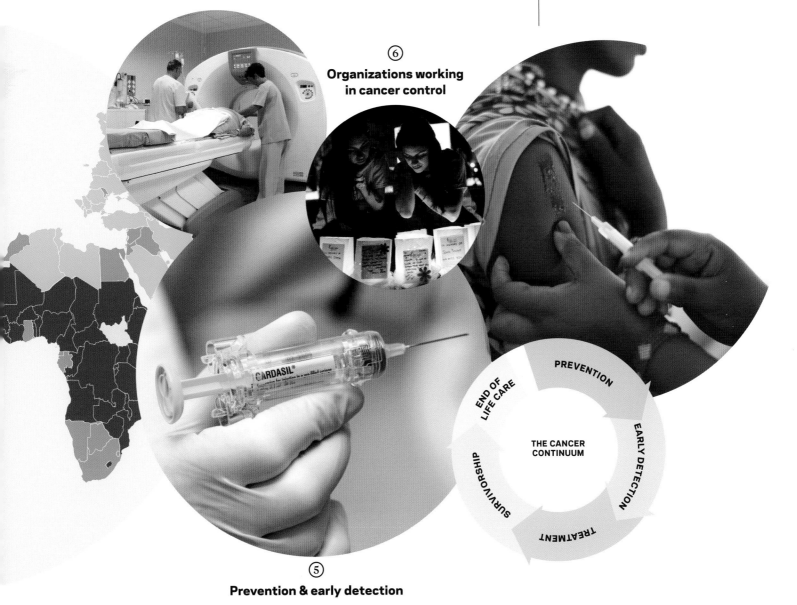

⑥
Organizations working in cancer control

THE CANCER CONTINUUM

PREVENTION

EARLY DETECTION

TREATMENT

SURVIVORSHIP

END OF LIFE CARE

⑤
Prevention & early detection

RISK
FACTORS

The growing prevalence of obesity and overweight, seen in every corner of the world, is the warning signal that big trouble is on its way.

— Margaret Chan, Director-General of the World Health Organization

Obesity

Worldwide, the number of overweight and obese (body mass index of 25 or greater) individuals increased from 857 million in 1980 to 2.1 billion in 2013.

NUMBER OF OVERWEIGHT AND OBESE INDIVIDUALS.

100 MILLION PEOPLE

1980
857,000,000

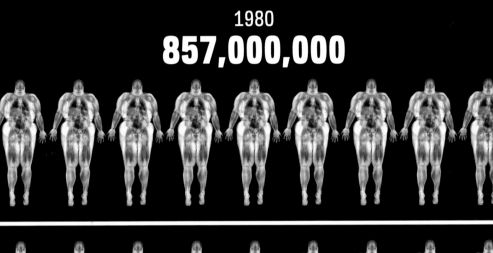

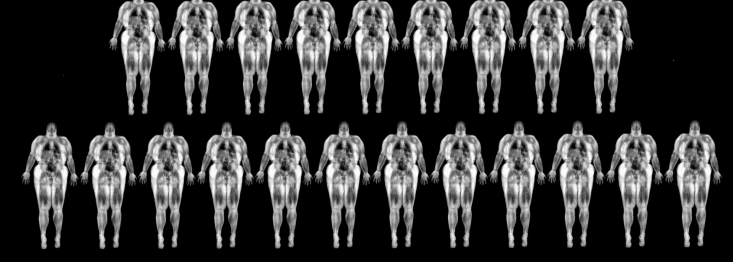

2013
2,100,000,000

OVERVIEW OF RISK FACTORS

Cancer can be caused by a variety of known risk factors, many of them preventable.

ENVIRONMENT

Cancer is mainly an environmental disease, as evidence in migrants suggests, with changes in risk that match those found in their new environment, sometimes even in first-generation immigrants. The *IARC World Cancer Report* addresses a number of risk factors for cancer.

①

Cancer is more often caused by the environment a person lives in, rather than his or her innate biology.

CANCER INCIDENCE AGE-STANDARDIZED RATES (WORLD) PER 100,000, CIRCA 1970

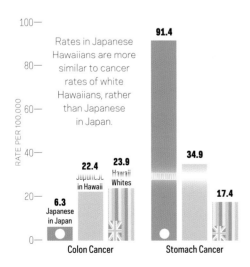

Rates in Japanese Hawaiians are more similar to cancer rates of white Hawaiians, rather than Japanese in Japan.

RATE PER 100,000

Colon Cancer: Japanese in Japan 6.3, Japanese in Hawaii 22.4, Hawaii Whites 23.9

Stomach Cancer: 91.4, 34.9, 17.4

TOBACCO

An estimated 1.3 billion people worldwide currently smoke tobacco, with the vast majority of these people smoking manufactured cigarettes. All forms of tobacco are carcinogenic; smoking causes over 16 types of cancer and accounts for about one-fifth of global cancer deaths. Nearly 40% of the reductions in male cancer death rates between 1991 and 2003 in the USA are thought to be attributed to smoking declines in the last half-century.

Smoking accounts for more than **20% of all cancer deaths worldwide.**

Lungs
Smokers are **15-30 times** more likely to get lung cancer than non-smokers.

Liver
Stomach
Pancreas
Kidneys
Ureter
Colorectum
Urinary bladder
Ovaries
Cervix

Smoking is associated with at least 16 types of cancers.

Nasal cavity and paranasal sinus
Oral cavity
Pharynx
Larynx
Esophagus
Bone marrow (acute myeloid leukemia)

INFECTIOUS AGENTS

According to a recent analysis, 16.1% of all cancers worldwide in 2008 were due to infectious agents. This fraction (the reduction in cancer if exposure to these infections was reduced to zero) was higher in less-developed countries (22.9%) than in more-developed countries (7.4%), and varied from 3.3% in Australia and New Zealand to 32.7% in sub-Saharan Africa.

OTHER RISK FACTORS

Other known risk factors include reproductive factors, environmental pollutants, and ultraviolet (UV) exposure. The extent of exposure to environmental carcinogenic pollutants is unknown, particularly in low-income countries, though the burden adds up to several hundred thousand newly diagnosed cancers per year just for arsenic, air pollution, affecting polychlorinated biphenyls and asbestos. Another environmental factor that is not man-made but is an important and preventable risk factor for skin cancer is excessive exposure to UV radiation, primarily from the sun, but also as a result of indoor tanning.

OCCUPATIONAL CARCINOGENS

The importance of occupational origin for a number of cancers, including mesothelioma, sinonasal, lung, nasopharynx, breast, non-melanoma skin cancer, bladder, esophagus, soft tissue sarcoma and stomach, has been highlighted in high-income countries. The carcinogens involved are asbestos, mineral oils, silica, diesel engine exhaust, coal tars and pitches, dioxins, environmental tobacco smoke, radon, tetrachloroethylene, arsenic and strong inorganic mists, and occupational exposures, including shift work, painting or welding. An emerging problem that needs to be addressed is that high-risk professions are now commonly exported to low-income countries.

③

Increasing intensity of occupational exposure to carcinogens carries increasing risk of developing cancer.

PERCENT OF MALES WHO DEVELOPED BLADDER CANCER BY OCCUPATIONAL EXPOSURE DURING THE MID-1900s

While a small proportion of the general male population will develop bladder cancer, the proportion of men who will develop bladder cancer increases with their increased intensity of exposure to occupational carcinogens. The observation by Case et al. that 100% of workers at distillers of beta-naphthylamine in the mid-1900s developed bladder cancer is a unique case in history.

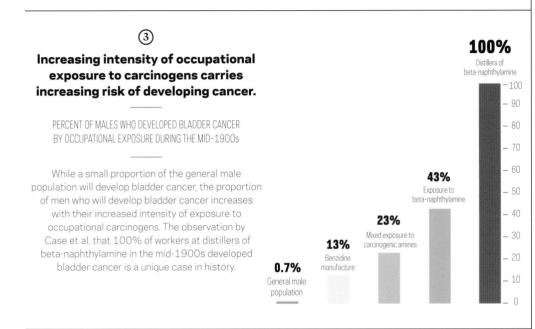

100%
Distillers of beta-naphthylamine

43%
Exposure to beta-naphthylamine

23%
Mixed exposure to carcinogenic amines

13%
Benzidine manufacture

0.7%
General male population

④

Compared with Northern America, the estimated prevalence of human papillomavirus (HPV), the leading cause of cervical cancer, is about three times as high in Europe and Latin America, and four times as high in Africa.

ESTIMATED HPV PREVALENCE (%), ALL TYPES COMBINED, AMONG WOMEN BY REGION, 1995-2009

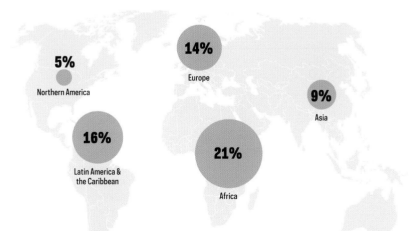

5% Northern America

14% Europe

9% Asia

16% Latin America & the Caribbean

21% Africa

Human papillomavirus types 16 and 18 are the most prevalent types of HPV worldwide, accounting for over 70% of all cervical cancer cases.

DIET

Obesity is a risk factor for breast (post-menopausal), colorectal, endometrial, kidney, esophageal and pancreatic cancers, though the burden of such diseases explained by diet, weight, and body fat is still uncertain. Alcohol use is clearly associated with liver, aero-digestive tract, breast and colorectal cancers. Dietary recommendations on dietary cancer prevention have been issued by the World Cancer Research Fund.

Dietary recommendations from the WCRF/AICR

The World Cancer Research Fund (WCRF/AICR) has released (and periodically updates) guidelines for cancer prevention:

1.
Be as lean as possible without becoming underweight.

2.
Be physically active for at least 30 minutes every day.

3.
Avoid sugary drinks.
Limit consumption of energy-dense foods (particularly processed foods high in added sugar, low in fiber, or high in fat).

4.
Eat a variety of vegetables, fruits, whole grains, and pulses such as beans.

5.
Limit consumption of red meats (such as beef, pork and lamb) and avoid processed meats.

6.
Limit alcoholic drinks to 2 drinks per day for men and 1 drink per day for women.

7.
Limit consumption of salty foods and foods processed with salt (sodium).

8.
Don't use supplements to protect against cancer. Instead, choose a balanced diet with a variety of foods.

RISKS OF TOBACCO

If current trends continue, approximately 1 billion people will die during the 21st century because of tobacco use.

Tobacco contains a wide range of harmful substances as well as a powerfully addictive drug, nicotine. ① Smoking tobacco significantly increases the risks of numerous cancers, including lung, esophagus, oral cavity, pharynx, and larynx. Smoking is also associated with many diseases other than cancer. By 2030, tobacco is projected to kill 8 million people annually.

While cigarette consumption is decreasing in high-income countries, it is increasing in many low- and middle-income countries. Between 1990 and 2009, for example, cigarette consumption decreased by 26% in Western Europe, while it increased by 57% in the Middle East and Africa. ② At the same time, few smokers in low- and middle-income countries are quitting smoking by middle age, when quitting can avoid more than 60% of the risk of lung cancer. ③ Where smoking prevalence is increasing, females may account for more of the increase than males.

In high-income countries, non-traditional tobacco products such as snus, lozenges, and chewing tobacco are promoted as alternatives in smoke-free environments or smoking cessation aids, but they are unsafe or have unknown effects. For example, smokeless tobacco causes cancer of the oral cavity, esophagus, and pancreas. Initial laboratory analyses of e-cigarettes found carcinogens and toxic chemicals in some samples. However, more research is needed before their harm or benefit can be accurately determined.

Non-smokers exposed to environmental tobacco smoke are also at increased risk of lung cancer and possibly other cancers. Secondhand smoke is estimated to cause 21,400 lung cancer deaths worldwide each year.

Lung cancer is highly fatal. In order to reduce these deaths, countries must work to prevent initiation of tobacco use in young people and encourage current smokers to quit.

①
Preventable deaths: a substantial proportion of cancer deaths are caused by tobacco, especially among men.

CANCER DEATHS (IN MILLIONS)
ATTRIBUTABLE TO TOBACCO, 2010

■ Cancer deaths attributable to tobacco

■ Other causes

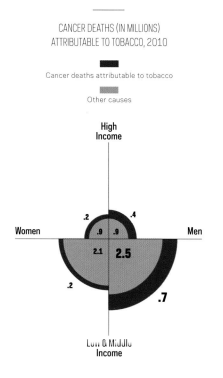

High Income

Women | Men

.2 | .4
.9 | .9
2.1 | 2.5
.2
.7

Low & Middle Income

②
Few smokers in low- and medium-Human Development Index (HDI) countries are quitting by middle age.

PERCENTAGE OF FORMER DAILY SMOKERS AMONG MEN AGE 45–54
BY HUMAN DEVELOPMENT INDEX (HDI)

◄ WEST | EAST ►

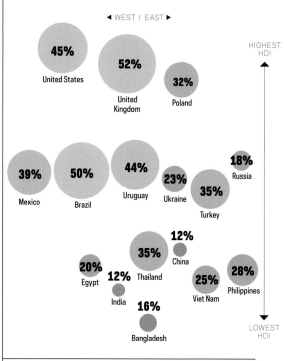

HIGHEST HDI

45% United States
52% United Kingdom
32% Poland

39% Mexico
50% Brazil
44% Uruguay
23% Ukraine
18% Russia
35% Turkey

20% Egypt
12% India
35% Thailand
12% China
16% Bangladesh
25% Viet Nam
28% Philippines

LOWEST HDI

The waterpipe, which features flavored tobacco smoked in a communal setting, has become popular among youth and young adults, and its use is increasing in many Global Youth Tobacco Survey countries.

In Lebanon, 25% of students reported smoking the waterpipe.

③
Smoking prevalence among girls is similar to or greater than that among adult women in many countries, indicating a potential future increase in the prevalence of smoking among women.

YOUTH AND ADULT SMOKING PREVALENCE

■ Youth ■ Adult

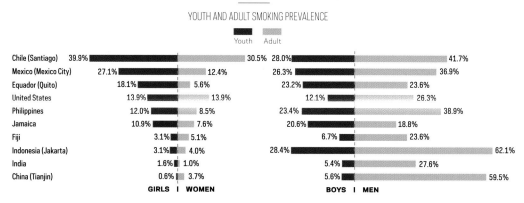

	GIRLS	WOMEN	BOYS	MEN
Chile (Santiago)	39.9%	30.5%	28.0%	41.7%
Mexico (Mexico City)	27.1%	12.4%	26.3%	36.9%
Equador (Quito)	18.1%	5.6%	23.2%	23.6%
United States	13.9%	13.9%	12.1%	26.3%
Philippines	12.0%	8.5%	23.4%	38.9%
Jamaica	10.9%	7.6%	20.6%	18.8%
Fiji	3.1%	5.1%	6.7%	23.6%
Indonesia (Jakarta)	3.1%	4.0%	28.4%	62.1%
India	1.6%	1.0%	5.4%	27.6%
China (Tianjin)	0.6%	3.7%	5.6%	59.5%

Prevalence of smoking among adults by sex

PERCENT, 2013

10.0% or less	10.1 — 20.0%	20.1 — 30.0%	30.1 — 40.0%	40.1 — 50.0%	50.1% or more	No Data

"If we do not act decisively, one hundred years from now our children and grandchildren will look back and seriously question how people claiming to be committed to public health and social justice allowed the tobacco epidemic to unfold unchecked."

—Dr. Gro Harlem Brundtland, Former Director-General WHO, Kobe, Japan, November 1999

Male

Female

INFECTION

Helicobacter pylori, HPV, HBV and HCV are important cancer-causing infectious agents.

"

"Viruses have had a checkered history in cancer biology over the past century. Depending on the time and the fashion, viruses have been either sought out as the primary cause for cancer, or ignored as inconsequential to this disease. We are now entering a more mature phase of research with the realization that a considerable proportion of cancers are indeed caused by viruses."

— Patrick S. Moore and Yuan Chang,
discoverers of the cancer-causing viruses Kaposi sarcoma-
associated herpesvirus and Merkel cell polyomavirus

① Worldwide, infectious agents are responsible for an estimated 2 million new cancer cases annually (16.1% of all cancers). The burden of these infection-related cancers is much higher in less-developed regions (22.9% overall and 32.7% in sub-Saharan Africa) versus more-developed regions (7.4%). The four main cancer-causing infectious agents—*Helicobacter pylori*, human papillomavirus, and hepatitis B and C viruses— are responsible for most infection-related cancers globally (mainly gastric, cervical and liver cancers, respectively).

Infection with the bacterium *Helicobacter pylori* is responsible for nearly 90% of stomach cancers worldwide and approximately 33% of all infection-related cancers. ② The prevalence of infection is especially common in less-developed regions, although it has been declining in recent generations.

Human papillomavirus (HPV) causes 28% of all infection-related cancers globally. Persistent HPV infection is responsible for nearly all cervical cancers, and a number of other cancers: vulvar (43%), vaginal (70%), anal (88%), penile (50%), and oropharyngeal (26% worldwide but more than 50% in North America, Australia, and Northern Europe). Although there are over 100 HPV types, HPV types 16 and 18 cause approximately 70% all of cervical cancers and about 90% of other HPV-related cancers. Cervical cancer remains a leading cause of cancer deaths among women in many less-developed regions of the world, where screening and treatment is often limited or unavailable.

Chronic infections with hepatitis B virus (HBV) and/or hepatitis C virus (HCV) account for more than 75% of liver cancers and 28% of all infection-related cancers. These infections are the most common infectious cause of cancer among men in less-developed regions of the world. HCV infection also causes some cases of non-Hodgkin lymphoma.

Less-common infections that cause cancer include Epstein-Barr virus, Kaposi sarcoma-associated herpesvirus, human T-cell lymphotropic virus, liver flukes, and schistosomal infections. Human immunodeficiency virus (HIV) infection also causes some cancers indirectly, especially infection-related cancers. Future research will likely identify both additional infections that cause cancer and more cancers associated with known infections.

Global transitions associated with development (including sanitation) and primary prevention including HBV and HPV vaccinations may decrease the infection-related cancer burden. Prevention is key to tackling the increasing cancer burden, particularly for low- and middle-income countries with weak health systems. Treatments for *Helicobacter pylori* and HCV infections are available but not widely used due to, respectively, lack of demonstration of efficacy to prevent gastric cancer and high cost. There is a need to develop low-cost and low-technology prevention and treatment measures for use in resource-limited settings where infection-related cancers are most common.

---

①
Many of the most common cancers are at least partly attributable to infection.

PERCENTAGE OF NEW CANCER CASES CAUSED BY INFECTION AND TOTAL NUMBER OF NEW CASES

■ Not attributable to infection

■ Number of cases attributable to infection

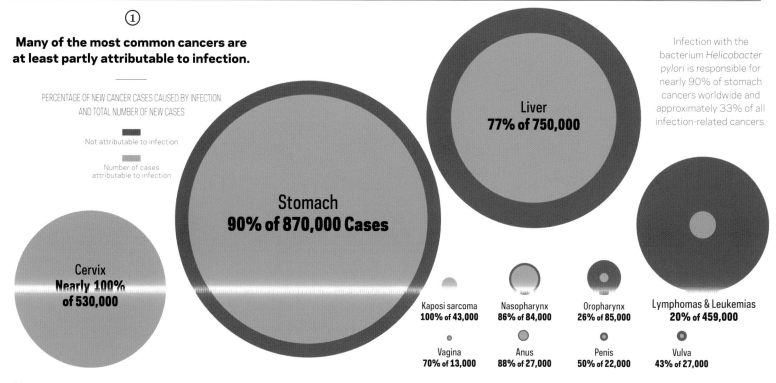

Stomach
90% of 870,000 Cases

Liver
77% of 750,000

Cervix
Nearly 100% of 530,000

Kaposi sarcoma
100% of 43,000

Nasopharynx
86% of 84,000

Oropharynx
26% of 85,000

Lymphomas & Leukemias
20% of 459,000

Vagina
70% of 13,000

Anus
88% of 27,000

Penis
50% of 22,000

Vulva
43% of 27,000

Infection with the bacterium *Helicobacter pylori* is responsible for nearly 90% of stomach cancers worldwide and approximately 33% of all infection-related cancers.

Fraction of new cancer cases attributable to infection

BY REGION, 2008

| 10.0% or less | 10.1—20.0% | 20.1—25.0% | 25.1—30.0% | 30.1% or more | No Data |

More-developed Regions ◄————————————————————► Less-developed Regions

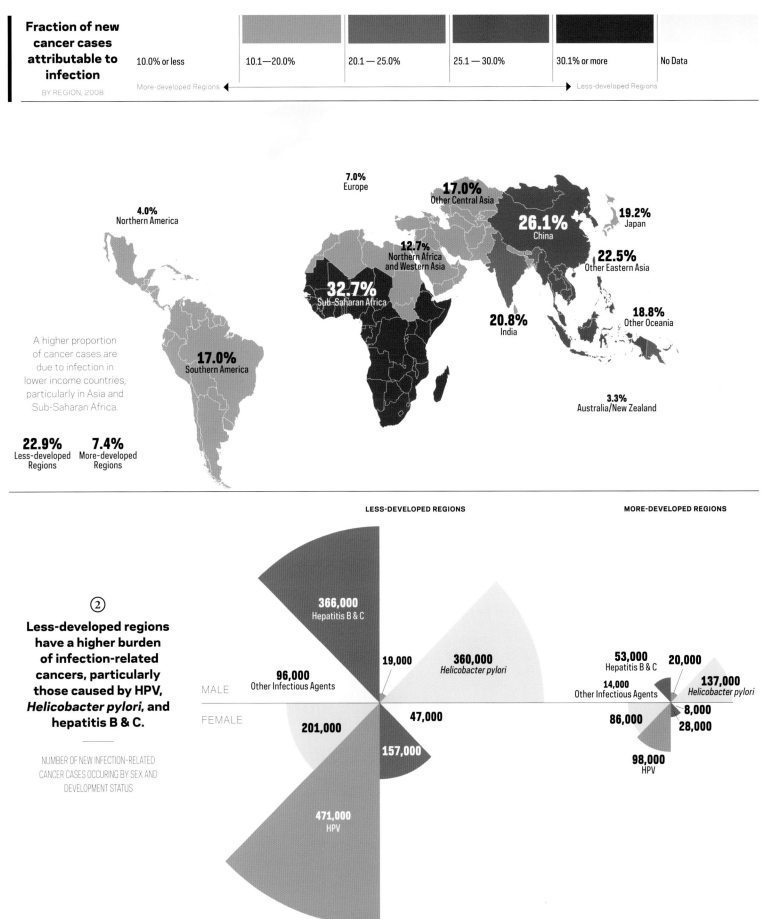

4.0% Northern America

7.0% Europe

17.0% Other Central Asia

26.1% China

19.2% Japan

12.7% Northern Africa and Western Asia

22.5% Other Eastern Asia

32.7% Sub-Saharan Africa

20.8% India

18.8% Other Oceania

17.0% Southern America

3.3% Australia/New Zealand

A higher proportion of cancer cases are due to infection in lower income countries, particularly in Asia and Sub-Saharan Africa.

22.9% Less-developed Regions

7.4% More-developed Regions

---

② **Less-developed regions have a higher burden of infection-related cancers, particularly those caused by HPV, *Helicobacter pylori*, and hepatitis B & C.**

NUMBER OF NEW INFECTION-RELATED CANCER CASES OCCURING BY SEX AND DEVELOPMENT STATUS

LESS-DEVELOPED REGIONS

MORE-DEVELOPED REGIONS

MALE

FEMALE

366,000 Hepatitis B & C

96,000 Other Infectious Agents

19,000

360,000 *Helicobacter pylori*

47,000

201,000

157,000

471,000 HPV

53,000 Hepatitis B & C

20,000

14,000 Other Infectious Agents

137,000 *Helicobacter pylori*

8,000

86,000

28,000

98,000 HPV

DIET, BODY MASS, AND PHYSICAL ACTIVITY

A healthy diet and body weight, together with recommended levels of physical activity, can significantly reduce the risk of developing and dying from cancer.

Poor diet, excess body weight, and physical inactivity are important risk factors for cancer. While research is ongoing to better understand the roles of these risk factors in cancer development, findings to date indicate that these factors can each individually affect cancer risk.

① A diet rich in plant foods such as fruits and non-starchy vegetables is associated with a lower risk of certain cancers. This type of diet also tends to be low in red and processed meats, which are associated with an increased risk of colorectal cancer. Alcohol increases the risk of cancer, and accounts for 4% of cancer deaths worldwide. In addition, dietary regimens and lifestyle factors can also have metabolic consequences (for example, hyperinsulinemia and inflammation), which could confer an increased risk of cancer.

② Overweight and obesity are associated with increased risk for certain cancers. Overweight and obesity are increasing in countries at all income levels. Emerging evidence also indicates that being overweight is associated with increased risk of cancer recurrence and decreased cancer survival.

Physical activity alone (regardless of body weight, diet, and other factors) is associated with reduced risk of certain cancers. Because physical activity helps prevent excess body weight, it also contributes to reduced risk of cancers associated with overweight and obesity. Thirty-one percent of adults worldwide do not meet the World Health Organization recommendation of 150 minutes of moderate physical activity or the equivalent each week.

While personal lifestyle choices can reduce the risk of cancer, governments and civil society also have a responsibility to develop food and economic policies conducive to health, create environments that support physical activity, and develop interventions targeting children and youth.

① Physical activity/inactivity and dietary factors can affect the risk of cancer.

STRENGTH OF EVIDENCE ON PHYSICAL ACTIVITY/INACTIVITY, DIETARY FACTORS, AND THE RISK OF CANCER

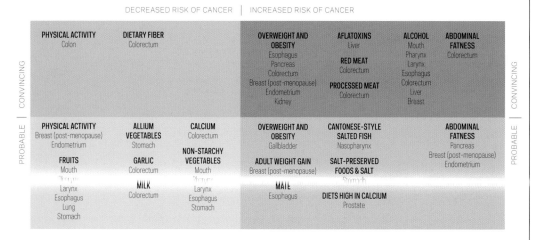

	DECREASED RISK OF CANCER		INCREASED RISK OF CANCER			
CONVINCING	PHYSICAL ACTIVITY Colon	DIETARY FIBER Colorectum		OVERWEIGHT AND OBESITY Esophagus Pancreas Colorectum Breast (post-menopause) Endometrium Kidney	AFLATOXINS Liver RED MEAT Colorectum PROCESSED MEAT Colorectum	ALCOHOL Mouth Pharynx Larynx Esophagus Colorectum Liver Breast	ABDOMINAL FATNESS Colorectum
PROBABLE	PHYSICAL ACTIVITY Breast (post-menopause) Endometrium FRUITS Mouth Pharynx Larynx Esophagus Lung Stomach	ALLIUM VEGETABLES Stomach GARLIC Colorectum MILK Colorectum	CALCIUM Colorectum NON-STARCHY VEGETABLES Mouth Pharynx Larynx Esophagus Stomach	OVERWEIGHT AND OBESITY Gallbladder ADULT WEIGHT GAIN Breast (post-menopause) MALE Esophagus	CANTONESE-STYLE SALTED FISH Nasopharynx SALT-PRESERVED FOODS & SALT Stomach DIETS HIGH IN CALCIUM Prostate		ABDOMINAL FATNESS Pancreas Breast (post-menopause) Endometrium

② For some cancer sites, excess body weight accounts for a large proportion of cases.

PERCENTAGE OF NEW CANCER CASES IN HIGH-INCOME COUNTRIES CAUSED BY EXCESS BODY WEIGHT

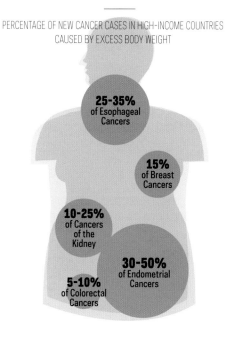

- 25-35% of Esophageal Cancers
- 15% of Breast Cancers
- 10-25% of Cancers of the Kidney
- 30-50% of Endometrial Cancers
- 5-10% of Colorectal Cancers

> "If we could give every individual the right amount of nourishment and exercise, not too little and not too much, we would have found the safest way to health."
>
> — *Hippocrates*

③ In some countries, physical inactivity accounts for a substantial proportion of colon cancer cases.

PERCENTAGE OF COLON CANCER CASES ATTRIBUTABLE TO PHYSICAL INACTIVITY

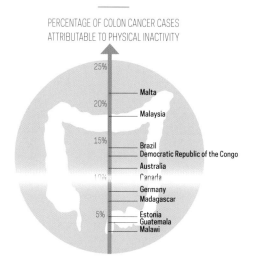

- 25%
- 20% — Malta
- — Malaysia
- 15% — Brazil
- — Democratic Republic of the Congo
- — Australia
- 10% — Canada
- — Germany
- — Madagascar
- 5% — Estonia
- — Guatemala
- — Malawi

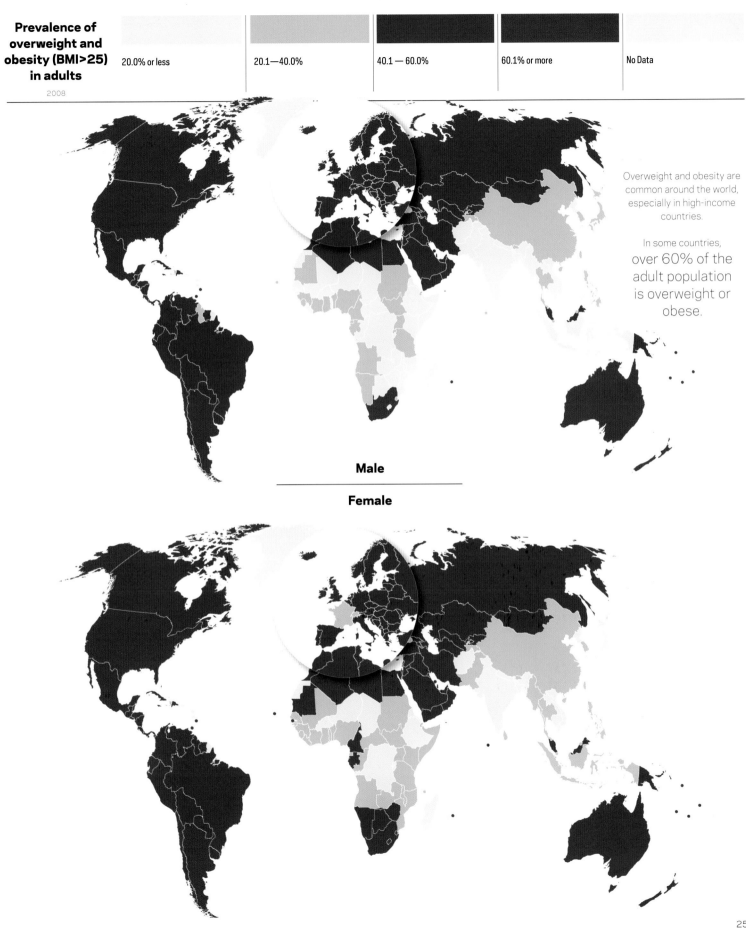

Prevalence of overweight and obesity (BMI>25) in adults

2008

| 20.0% or less | 20.1—40.0% | 40.1 — 60.0% | 60.1% or more | No Data |

Overweight and obesity are common around the world, especially in high-income countries.

In some countries, over 60% of the adult population is overweight or obese.

Male

Female

ULTRAVIOLET RADIATION

UV radiation exposure increases the risk of skin cancers, the most common cancers in humans. Sun protection reduces the risk of skin cancer.

Ultraviolet (UV) radiation is a major risk factor for melanoma of the skin. About 230,000 cases and 55,000 deaths from melanoma are estimated to occur each year worldwide. UV radiation also causes keratinocyte (also known as non-melanoma) skin cancers, the most common types of cancer in humans with about 13 million cases each year. ① While rarely fatal, keratinocyte cancers impose a significant burden of morbidity and economic cost.

The major source of UV radiation is the sun. The amount of solar radiation reaching any point on the Earth's surface depends on latitude and altitude, time of day and year, cloud cover, and air pollution; UV radiation levels also depend on the protective stratospheric ozone layer.

② Personal exposures to "artificial" UV radiation up to 10-15 times stronger than summer midday sun in Southern Europe may occur through the use of tanning devices. Although classified as a human carcinogen, they have been commonly used for cosmetic purposes.

In addition to ambient UV radiation and occupational and recreational sun exposure, other risk factors for skin cancer are fair skin color and sensitivity to the sun, which are inherited characteristics. People with innately dark skin have very low rates of skin cancer; those with light skin and hair, blue or green eyes, and many moles have much higher rates. The risk is also higher with high UV radiation exposure in childhood.

Sunscreens protect skin against UV radiation, but are only part of a sun-safe strategy, which also includes wearing sunglasses, hats and protective clothing; staying out of the sun in the middle part of the day; and providing effective shade structures for outdoor venues. Since 1983, Australia has been implementing skin cancer prevention campaigns based on this strategy. ③ While it will take many years to witness the full effects of this program, rates of melanoma are already decreasing among youth.

① Keratinocyte (nonmelanoma) skin cancer costs millions of dollars each year.

ESTIMATED ANNUAL COST OF KERATINOCYTE (NONMELANOMA) SKIN CANCERS IN US DOLLARS BY COST PER CASE AND TOTAL COST PER COUNTRY

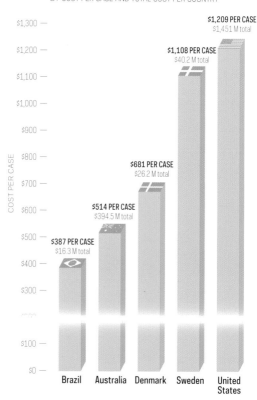

COST PER CASE

- **$387 PER CASE** $16.3 M total — Brazil
- **$514 PER CASE** $394.5 M total — Australia
- **$681 PER CASE** $26.2 M total — Denmark
- **$1,108 PER CASE** $40.2 M total — Sweden
- **$1,209 PER CASE** $1,451 M total — United States

② Both boys and girls in some countries use sunbeds, which increases the risk of developing skin cancer later in life.

PREVALENCE OF SUNBED USE AMONG YOUTH

Girls Boys

	Girls	Boys
United States Grades 9-12 (2009)	25%	7%
Canada Ages 16-24 (2006)	27%	8%
Sweden Ages 15-19 (1999)	45%	19%
Denmark Ages 15-19 (2007)	59%	42%

Use of sunbeds by young people is common in some countries. Prevalence = use at least once in past 12 months.

Incidence of melanoma of the skin in both sexes

ESTIMATED AGE-STANDARDIZED RATE (WORLD) PER 100,000 POPULATION, 2012

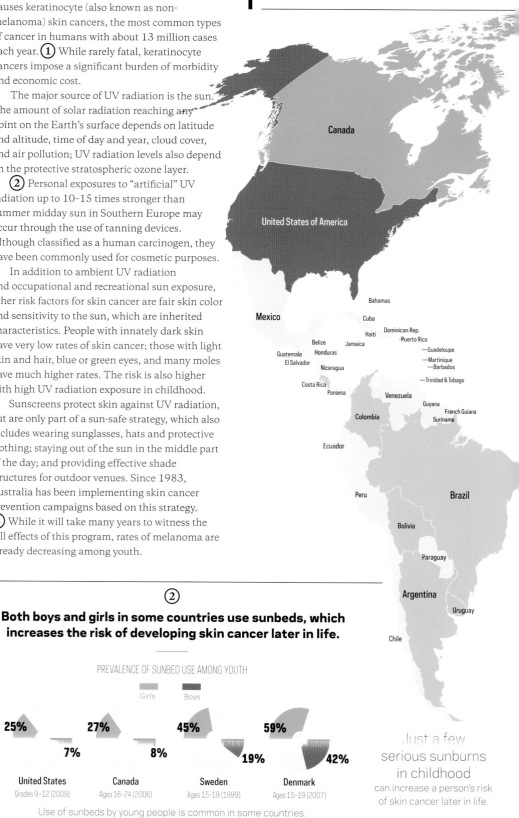

Just a few serious sunburns in childhood can increase a person's risk of skin cancer later in life.

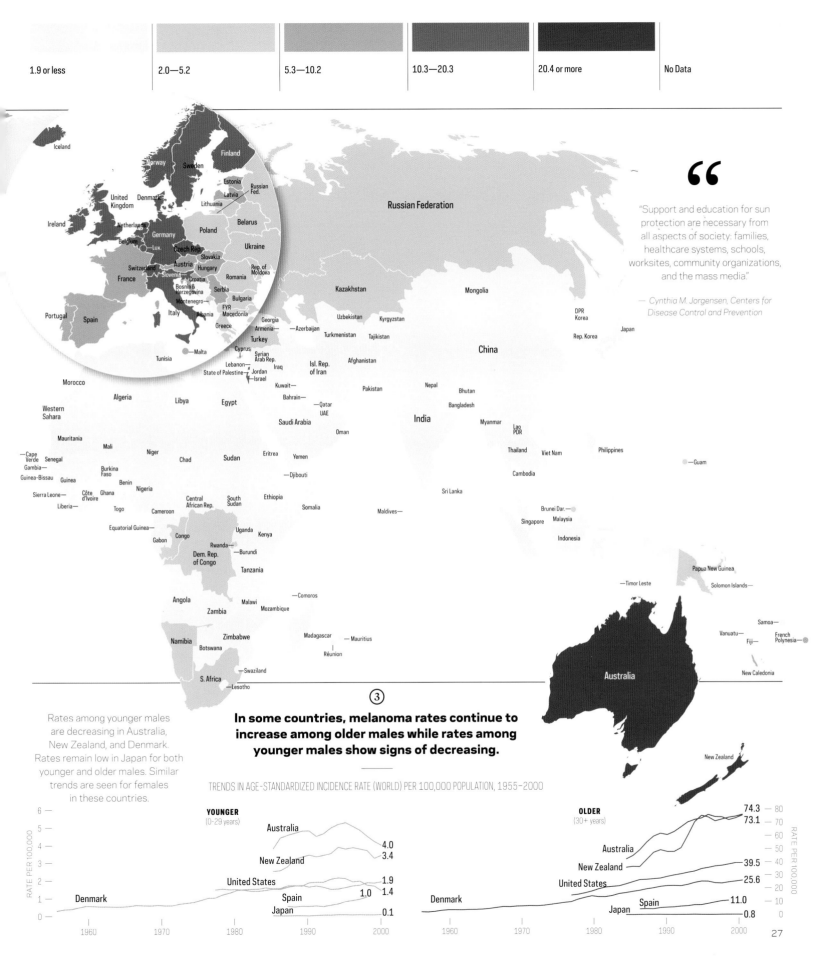

| 1.9 or less | 2.0—5.2 | 5.3—10.2 | 10.3—20.3 | 20.4 or more | No Data |

"Support and education for sun protection are necessary from all aspects of society: families, healthcare systems, schools, worksites, community organizations, and the mass media."

— *Cynthia M. Jorgensen, Centers for Disease Control and Prevention*

③

In some countries, melanoma rates continue to increase among older males while rates among younger males show signs of decreasing.

Rates among younger males are decreasing in Australia, New Zealand, and Denmark. Rates remain low in Japan for both younger and older males. Similar trends are seen for females in these countries.

TRENDS IN AGE-STANDARDIZED INCIDENCE RATE (WORLD) PER 100,000 POPULATION, 1955–2000

YOUNGER (0-29 years)

RATE PER 100,000

- Australia 4.0
- New Zealand 3.4
- United States 1.9
- Spain 1.0
- 1.4
- Japan 0.1

1960 1970 1980 1990 2000

OLDER (30+ years)

RATE PER 100,000

- Australia 74.3 / 73.1
- New Zealand 39.5
- United States 25.6
- Spain 11.0
- Japan 0.8

1960 1970 1980 1990 2000

REPRODUCTIVE AND HORMONAL FACTORS

Reproductive and hormonal factors have changed over the last century, resulting in changing risk patterns for associated cancers.

Reproductive habits and women's hormonal status have changed enormously over the past century. ① Age at menarche and the average number of births have decreased, mainly in high-income countries.

② Reproductive risk factors for female breast and endometrial cancer are related to the levels of estrogens in the body. Having menarche at a younger age increases the number of years the breast tissue is exposed to high levels of estrogens. ③ Women who have their first full-term pregnancy at an early age have a decreased risk of developing breast cancer later in life, probably due to increased differentiation of the breast epithelial cells. The risk also declines with the number of children borne, and with breastfeeding for at least a year. Late menopause also increases the risk of breast cancer by increasing the duration of breast exposure to estrogen. A number of studies have suggested that current use of oral contraceptives causes a small and transient increase in the risk of breast cancer. However, the use of oral contraceptives causes a long-term and substantial reduction in the risk of endometrial and ovarian cancers.

Menopausal hormone therapy, often prescribed for short-term benefits, such as relief from hot flashes, is associated with a moderate increase in the risk for certain cancers including breast cancer, and the risk for breast cancer is greater for treatments containing both an estrogen and a progestogen. An IARC Monographs Working Group has concluded that combined estrogen-progestogen oral contraceptives and combined estrogen-progestogen menopausal therapy are carcinogenic to humans.

---

①

Earlier age at menarche is associated with increased risk of certain cancers; during the twentieth century, age at menarche decreased in many high-income countries.

TRENDS IN AGE AT MENARCHE IN NORWAY AND THE USA

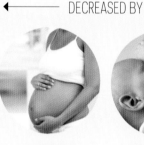

- 15—
- **14.6** **13.2** (Oslo, Norway) — 1918 / 1964
- **14.3** **12.5** (United States) — 1914 / 1970
- 12—
- 9—
- 6—
- 3—
- 0—

---

②

Breastfeeding and childbearing reduce the risk of breast cancer among women, whereas oral contraceptive use and hormone replacement therapy increase the risk.

HORMONAL AND REPRODUCTIVE RISK FACTORS FOR BREAST CANCER

← DECREASED BY ——   —— INCREASED BY →

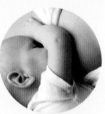
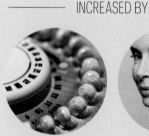
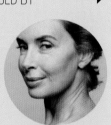

CHILDBEARING
About 7% lowered risk per child; having the first live birth after age 30 doubles the risk compared to having first live birth at age younger than 20

BREASTFEEDING
Decreases risk by 4.3% per breastfeeding year

ORAL CONTRACEPTIVES
Slight increase in current users

HORMONE REPLACEMENT THERAPY
Moderate increase in users for 5 or more years after menopause; larger with estrogen and progestogen than for estrogen alone

---

③

Larger family sizes and longer lifetime length of breastfeeding, while no longer representative of reproductive patterns in developed countries today, result in fewer cases of breast cancer.

ESTIMATED FEWER CASES OF BREAST CANCER WITH HYPOTHETICAL REPRODUCTIVE PATTERNS OF THE PAST, NUMBER OF CASES PER 100 70-YEAR-OLD WOMEN LIVING IN DEVELOPED COUNTRIES

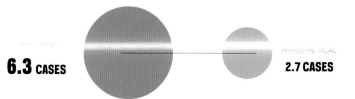

6.3 CASES   **2.7 CASES**
HYPOTHETICAL

Estimate based on an average of 2.5 children and 8.7 months breastfeeding in developed countries; "larger family sizes" are defined as an average of 6.5 children; longer durations of breastfeeding are defined as total of 13 years of breastfeeding.

Average number of children borne per woman

FERTILITY PER WOMAN, 1970-1975 AND 2005-2010

1.9 or fewer	2.0 — 2.9	3.0 — 4.3	4.4 — 5.8	5.9 — 7.4	7.5 — 8.5	No Data

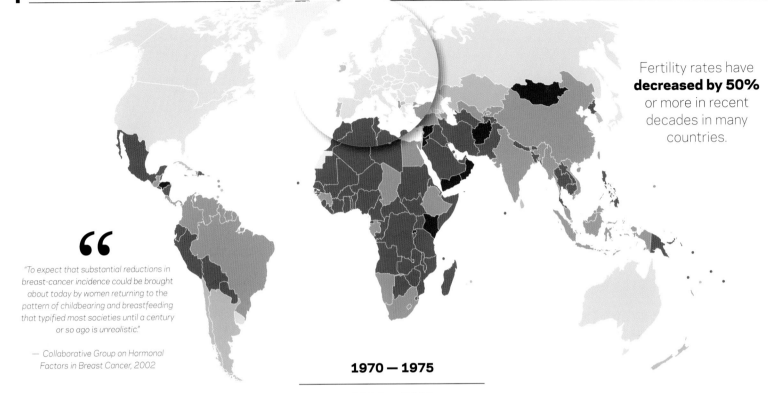

Fertility rates have **decreased by 50%** or more in recent decades in many countries.

> "To expect that substantial reductions in breast-cancer incidence could be brought about today by women returning to the pattern of childbearing and breastfeeding that typified most societies until a century or so ago is unrealistic."
>
> — Collaborative Group on Hormonal Factors in Breast Cancer, 2002

1970 — 1975

2005 — 2010

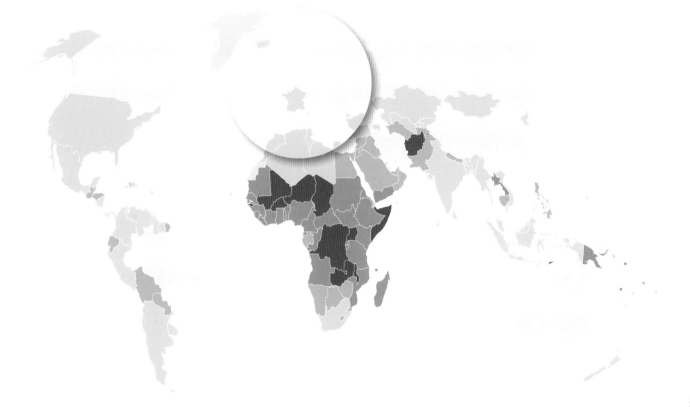

ENVIRONMENTAL & OCCUPATIONAL POLLUTANTS

Limiting carcinogenic exposures in the environment and in the workplace provides an opportunity to reduce the cancer burden, particularly for workers with unacceptable exposures.

ENVIRONMENTAL POLLUTANTS

Exposure to radon is the second leading cause of lung cancer in the USA and Europe. Radon gas forms from the radioactive decay of uranium, found at differing concentrations in soil and rock throughout the world. Exposure occurs when radon gas is trapped in underground mines and basements.

Populations consuming high levels of arsenic in drinking water have excess risks of skin, lung and bladder cancer. High levels of arsenic in drinking water have been found in areas in the People's Republic of China, Bangladesh, Taiwan (China), and some countries in Central and South America.

① Indoor air pollution from solid fuel use is estimated to cause about 2.5 million deaths each year in developing countries, or about 4.5% of global deaths annually. The International Agency for Research on Cancer (IARC) classifies indoor smoke emissions from coal as known human carcinogens, and from other types of solid fuels as probable carcinogens.

Exposure to fine particulate matter in outdoor air increases lung cancer risk. Outdoor air pollution levels are particularly high in rapidly growing cities in developing countries. Diesel exhaust, also classified as a lung carcinogen by IARC, contributes to outdoor air pollution and is also an occupational lung carcinogen.

② Many substances are known to cause cancer among exposed industrial workers.

IARC-CLASSIFIED GROUP I CARCINOGENS
FOR WHICH EXPOSURES ARE MOSTLY OCCUPATIONAL
(EXCLUDING PESTICIDES AND DRUGS), BY CANCER.

EXPOSURE	MAIN INDUSTRY/USE
BLADDER	
4-Aminobiphenyl (92-67-1)	Rubber manufacture
Coal tar pitches (65996-93-2)	Building material, electrodes
2-Naphthylamine (91-59-8)	Dye/pigment manufacture
Benzidine (92-87-5)	Dye/pigment manufacture, laboratory agent
LUNG	
Beryllium (7440-41-7) and beryllium compounds	Aerospace industry/metals
Bis(chloromethyl) ether (542-88-11)	Chemical intermediate/by-product
Chloromethyl methyl ether (107-30-2) (technical grade)	
Cadmium (7440-43-9) and cadmium compounds	Dye/pigment manufacture
Talc containing asbestiform fibers	Paper, paints
LEUKEMIA	
Benzene (71-43-2)	Solvent, fuel
Ethylene oxide (75-21-8)	Chemical intermediate, sterilant
NASAL CAVITY	
Wood dust	Wood industry
SKIN	
Mineral oils, untreated and mildly treated	Lubricants
Shale oils (68308-34-9)	Lubricants, fuels
PHARYNX, LUNG	
Mustard gas (sulphur mustard) (505-60-2)	War gas
NASAL CAVITY, LUNG	
Chromium (VI) compounds	Metal plating, dye/pigment manufacture
Nickel compounds	Metallurgy, alloys, catalyst
SKIN, LUNG	
Coal tars (8007-45-2)	Fuel
Arsenic (7440-38-2) and arsenic compounds	Glass, metals, pesticides
Soots	Pigments
SKIN, LUNG, BLADDER	
Coal tar pitches (65996-93-2)	Building material, electrodes
LIVER, LUNG, BLOOD VESSELS	
Vinyl chloride (75-01-4)	Plastics, monomer
LUNG, PLEURA, PERITONEUM	
Asbestos (1332-21-4)	Insulation, filter material, textiles

①

Indoor air pollution from use of solid fuels for heating or cooking, mostly in lower-income countries, is estimated to cause about 4 million deaths each year worldwide.

POPULATION USING SOLID FUELS (%), 2010

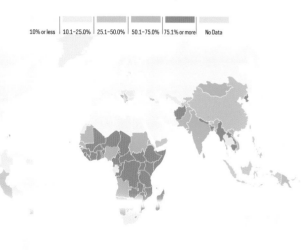

10% or less | 10.1–25.0% | 25.1–50.0% | 50.1–75.0% | 75.1% or more | No Data

Exposure to particulate matter

ANNUAL MEAN LEVEL OF PM2.5 (PARTICULATE MATTER OF 2.5 μm DIAMETER OR LESS) MEASURED IN μg/m³, 2008-2013

14.4 or less	14.5—25.5	25.6—41.3	41.4—64.1	64.2 or more	No Data

"The air we breathe has become polluted with a mixture of cancer-causing substances. We now know that outdoor air pollution is not only a major risk to health in general, but also a leading environmental cause of cancer deaths."

— Dr. Kurt Straif, Head of the IARC Monographs Section

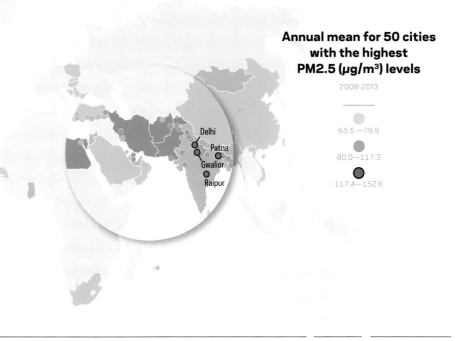

Annual mean for 50 cities with the highest PM2.5 (μg/m³) levels

2008-2013

- 65.5 —79.9
- 80.0—117.3
- 117.4—152.6

Delhi
Patna
Gwalior
Raipur

OCCUPATIONAL EXPOSURES

(2) Numerous substances in the workplace are known to cause cancer in workers, as are certain work circumstances. Due to the intensity and/or duration of these exposures, the cancer burden can be quite high among those workers exposed. Though preventing these cancers is possible where steps can be taken to limit exposure, occupational exposure remains a particular concern in low- and middle-income countries, where exposures are likely to be higher, regulations and enforcement are less strict than in high-income countries, and hazardous exposures occur in small-scale industrial operations.

(3) For example, asbestos, used in industrialized countries for insulation, friction products, and fire protection until the 1980s, is an important cause of occupational lung cancer and the unique cause of malignant mesothelioma, a rare and lethal cancer. (4) Asbestos exposure remains an occupational and environmental hazard in many countries.

* The top 7 Western European consumers in 1970: UK, Italy, W. Germany, E. Germany, France, Spain, and Belgium/Luxembourg. Includes E. Germany so that the number for 2003 is comparable.
** USSR for 1970; Russia and Kazakhstan for 2003.

(3)

Asbestos is a known cause of a rare, lethal type of lung cancer known as mesothelioma.

TONS OF ASBESTOS USED 1920-1970 AND MESOTHELIOMA DEATHS 1994-2008

	TONS ASBESTOS (MILLIONS) 1920-1970	MESOTHELIOMA DEATHS 1994-2008
USA	21.8 ▶	36,600
United Kingdom	4.8 ▶	28,400
Germany	4.1 ▶	16,000
Japan	3.2 ▶	12,000
France	2.3 ▶	12,400

(4)

Asbestos consumption has dramatically declined in many countries, but has remained the same or increased in some fast-growing economies.

ASBESTOS CONSUMPTION IN SELECTED COUNTRIES/REGIONS, 1970 VS. 2003

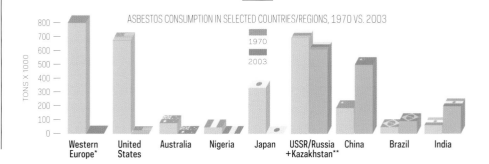

1970
2003

TONS X 1000

Western Europe* · United States · Australia · Nigeria · Japan · USSR/Russia +Kazakhstan** · China · Brazil · India

HUMAN CARCINOGENS IDENTIFIED BY THE IARC MONOGRAPHS PROGRAM

To date, IARC has classified over 100 agents as carcinogenic to humans.

The IARC Monographs (*www.monographs.iarc.fr*) identify environmental and occupational causes of human cancer. Sometimes called the WHO "Encyclopedia of Carcinogens," the IARC Monographs are critical reviews and evaluations of the weight of the evidence that an agent can increase the risk of cancer in humans. Since its inception in 1971, some 1000 agents have been evaluated, including individual chemicals, complex mixtures, physical agents, biological agents, personal habits, and occupational exposures.

The agents are classified as "carcinogenic to humans" (Group 1), "probably carcinogenic to humans" (Group 2A), "possibly carcinogenic to humans" (Group 2B), "not classifiable as to their carcinogenicity to humans" (Group 3), or as "probably not carcinogenic to humans" (Group 4). This classification, based on all available scientific literature, reflects the strength of the evidence derived from epidemiological studies in humans, cancer bioassays in experimental animals, and in-vivo and in-vitro studies on the mechanisms of carcinogenicity. The studies in humans and in experimental animals are considered as providing sufficient evidence, limited evidence, inadequate evidence, or evidence suggesting lack of carcinogenicity. Data from mechanistic studies are considered as providing strong, moderate, or weak evidence

for a given mechanism. To date, over 100 agents have been classified in Group 1, the vast majority on the basis of sufficient evidence from epidemiological studies that the agent can cause cancer at one or several sites in humans. Nevertheless, some important risk factors widely known to cause cancer in humans, such as obesity or reproductive factors for breast cancer, have not been evaluated by the Monographs program.

The main figure shows, for each organ or group of organs in the human body, which agent(s) can cause an increased risk of cancer at a given site. Over 40 agents have more than one organ site, with up to 17 sites for tobacco smoking and 14 sites for X-radiation and gamma-radiation. Some agents have been classified in Group 1 with less than sufficient evidence from epidemiological studies (no target organ identified), often on the basis of sufficient evidence of carcinogenicity in experimental animals and strong evidence in exposed humans that the agent acts through a relevant mechanism of carcinogenicity. It is noteworthy that a few agents have been shown to cause cancer in the offspring of the person exposed.

Agents without a Target Site

Areca nut
Aristolochic acid
Benzidine, dyes metabolized to Benzo(a)pyrene
Ethanol in alcoholic beverages
Ethylene oxide
Etoposide
Ionizing radiation (all types)
4, 4'-Methylenebis (2-chloroaniline) (MOCA)
Neutron radiation
N'-Nitrosonornicotine, (NNN) and 4-(N-nitroso-methyl-amino-1-(3-pyridyl)-1-butnone (NNK)

2,3,4,7,8-Pentachlorodibenzofuran
3,4,5,3',4'- Pentachlorobiphenyl (PCB-126)
Polychlorinated biphenyls dioxin-lke, with a Toxic Equivalent Factor according to WHO (PCBs 77, 81, 105, 114, 118, 123, 126, 156, 167,169, 189)
Radionuclides, alpha-particle emitting, internally deposited
Radionuclides, beta-paticle emitting, internalldeposited,
Ultraviolet radiation

Multiple or All Sites

MULTIPLE SITES (UNSPECIFIED)
CyclosporineFission products, including Strontium-90
X-ray gamma-radiation (exposure in utero)

ALL CANCERS COMBINED
2,3,7,8-Tetrachlorodibenzo-para-dioxin

Endothelium (Kaposi Sarcoma)

Human immunodeficiency virus type 1
Kaposi sarcoma herpes-virus

① Brain and Central Nervous System

X-ray, gamma-radiation

② Eye

Human immunodeficiency virus type 1
Ultraviolet-emitting tanning devices
Welding

③ Oral Cavity and Pharynx

ORAL CAVITY	PHARYNX (ORO-, HYPO- AND/OR NOT OTHERWISE SPECIFIED)
Alcoholic beverages	Alcoholic beverages
Betel quid with tobacco	Betel quid with tobacco
Betel quid without tobacco	Human papillomavirus type 16
Human papillomavirus type 16	Tobacco smoking
Smokeless tobacco	
Tobacco smoking	

TONSIL	NASOPHARYNX
Human papillomavirus type 16	Epstein-Barr virus
	Formaldehyde
SALIVARY GLAND	Salted fish, Chinese-style
X-ray, gamma-radiation	Wood dust

④ Respiratory System

NASAL CAVITY AND PARANASAL SINUS	LARYNX
Isopropyl alcohol manufacture using strong acids	Acid mists, strong inorganic
Leather dust	Alcoholic beverages
Nickel compounds	Asbestos (all forms)
Radium-226 and its decay products	Tobacco smoking
Radium-228 and its decay products	**PLEURA OR PERITONEUM (MESOTHELIOMA)**
Tobacco smoking	Asbestos (all forms)
Wood dust	Erionite
	Painter (occupational exposure as)

LUNG

Aluminum production	Iron and steel founding
Arsenic and inorganic arsenic compounds	MOPP (vincristine-prednisone-nitrogen mustard-procarbazine mixture)
Asbestos (all forms)	Nickel compounds
Beryllium and beryllium compounds	Outdoor air pollution
Bis(chloromethyl)ether; chloromethyl methyl ether (technical grade)	Outdoor air pollution, particulate matter in
Cadmium and cadmium compounds	Painter (occupational exposure as)
Chromium (VI) compounds	Plutonium
Coal, indoor emissions from household combustion	Radon-222 and its decay products
Coal gasification	Rubber production industry
Coal-tar pitch	Silica dust, crystalline
Coke production	Soot
Diesel engine exhausts	Sulfur mustard
Hematite mining (underground)	Tobacco smoke, secondhand
	Tobacco smoking
	X-ray, gamma-radiation

CARCINOGENIC AGENTS BY TARGET SITE*

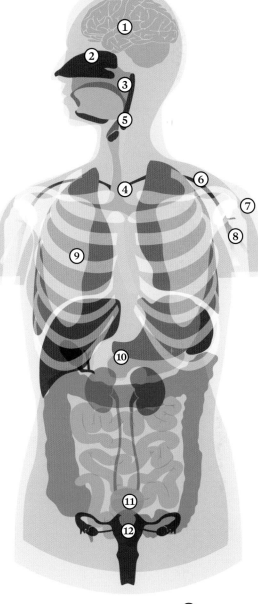

⑤ Thyroid

Radioiodines, including iodine-131
(exposure during childhood and adolescence)

X-ray, gamma-radiation

⑥ Hematopoietic System

Azathioprine
Benzene
Busulfan
1,3-Butadiene
Chlorambucil
Cyclophosphamide
Cyclosporine
Epstein-Barr virus
Etoposide with cisplatin and bleomycin
Fission products, including Strontium-90
Formaldehyde
Helicobacter pylori
Hepatitis C virus
Human immunodeficiency virus type 1
Human T-cell lymphotropic virus type 1

Kaposi sarcoma herpes virus
Melphalan
MOPP (vincristine-prednisone-nitrogen mustard-procarbazine mixture)
Phosphorus-32, as phosphate
Rubber production industry
Semustine [1-(2-Chloroethyl)-3-(4-methylcyclohexyl)-1-nitrosourea, or methyl-CCNU]
Thiotepa
Thorium-232 and its decay products
Tobacco smoking
Treosulfan
X-ray, gamma-radiation

⑦ Skin

OTHER MALIGNANT NEOPLASMS
Arsenic and inorganic arsenic compounds
Azathioprine
Coal-tar distillation
Coal-tar pitch
Cyclosporine
Methoxsalen plus ultraviolet A
Mineral oils, untreated or mildly treated
Shale oils
Solar radiation
Soot
X-ray, gamma-radiation

MELANOMA
Solar radiation
Polychlorinated biphenyls
Ultraviolet-emitting tanning devices

⑧ Bone

Plutonium
Radium-224 and its decay products
Radium-226 and its decay products
Radium-228 and its decay products
X-ray, gamma-radiation

⑨ Breast

Alcoholic beverages
Diethylstilbestrol
Estrogen-progestogen contraceptives
Estrogen-progestogen menopausal therapy
X-ray, gamma-radiation

⑩ Digestive System

ESOPHAGUS
Acetaldehyde associated with consumption of alcoholic beverages
Alcoholic beverages
Betel quid with tobacco
Betel quid without tobacco
Smokeless tobacco
Tobacco smoking
X-ray, gamma-radiation

UPPER AERODIGESTIVE TRACT
Acetaldehyde associated with consumption of alcoholic beverages

STOMACH
Helicobacter pylori
Rubber production industry
Tobacco smoking
X-radiation, gamma-radiation

COLON AND RECTUM
Alcoholic beverages
Tobacco smoking
X-ray, gamma-radiation

ANUS
Human immunodefefiency virus type 1
Human papillomavirus 16

LIVER (HEPATOCELLULAR CARCINOMA)
Aflatoxins
Alcoholic beverages
Estrogen-progestogen contraceptives
Hepatitis B virus
Hepatitis C virus
Plutonium
Thorium-232 and its decay products
Tobacco smoking (in smokers and in smokers' children)

LIVER (ANGIOSARCOMA)
Vinyl chloride

BILIARY TRACT
Chlonorchis sinensis
Opisthorchis viverrini

GALLBLADDER
Thorium-232 and its decay products

PANCREAS
Smokeless tobacco
Tobacco smoking

⑪ Urinary System

KIDNEY
Tobacco smoking
Trichloroethylene
X-ray, gamma-radiation

RENAL PELVIS
Aristolochic acid, plants containing Phenacetin
Phenacetin, analgesic mixtures containing
Tobacco smoking

URETER
Aristolochic acid, plants containing Phenacetin
Phenacetin, analgesic mixtures containing
Tobacco smoking

URINARY BLADDER
Aluminum production
4-Aminobiphenyl
Arsenic and inorganic arsenic compounds
Auramine production
Benzidine
Chlornaphazine
Cyclophosphamide
Magenta production
2-Naphthylamine
Painter (occupational exposure as)
Rubber production industry
Schistosoma haematobium
Tobacco smoking
ortho-Toluidine
X-ray, gamma-radiation

⑫ Genital System

CERVIX
Diethylstilbestrol (exposure in utero)
Estrogen-progestogen contraceptives
Human immunodeficiency virus type 1
Human papillomavirus types 16, 18, 31, 33, 35, 39, 45, 51, 52, 56, 58, 59
Tobacco smoking

ENDOMETRIUM
Estrogen menopausal therapy
Estrogen-progestogen menopausal therapy
Tamoxifen

OVARY
Asbestos (all forms)
Estrogen menopausal therapy
Tobacco smoking

VAGINA
Diethylstilbestrol (exposure in utero)
Human papillomavirus type 16

VULVA
Human papillomavirus type 16

PENIS
Human papillomavirus type 16

*Target sites are numbered by anatomic placement and not by number of carcinogens associated with the site or impact of carcinogens on disease burden.

THE
BURDEN

"

Cancer, already the leading cause
of death in many high-income
countries, is set to become a major
cause of morbidity and mortality
in the next few decades in every
region of the world, irrespective
of level of resource.

— *Bray F et al.*, Lancet Oncology,
2012

Growth of New Cancer Cases

The annual number of new cancer cases in the world is predicted to increase from over 14 million in 2012 to almost 22 million in 2030 due to population growth and aging alone. The biggest increases of 70% will be seen in Africa, Asia and Latin America, which include many countries that lack adequate resources to deal with the rising number of cancer patients.

500,000 CASES

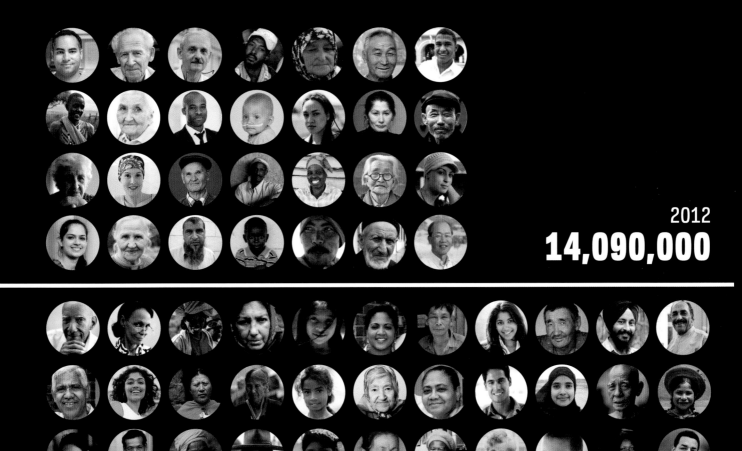

2012
14,090,000

2030
21,681,000

THE BURDEN OF CANCER

Cancer, as a group, represents the most important cause of death worldwide, with the number of deaths exceeding that for ischemic heart disease or any other specific disease grouping.

The risk of developing cancer before 75 years can approach 35% (over 1 in 3) in some countries. ① Worldwide, there were an estimated 14.1 million new cancer cases and 8.2 million cancer deaths in 2012. Of these, 57% (8 million) of new cancer cases and 65% (5.3 million) of the cancer deaths occurred in the less-developed regions of the world. Almost half of all new cancer cases and slightly more than half of all cancer deaths occur in Asia, and one quarter of the global burden occurs in China.

By the year 2025, there will be an estimated 19.3 million new cancer cases and 11.4 million cancer deaths, and the proportions of these occurring in less-developed regions will increase to 59% and 68% respectively.

② Lung and prostate cancers are the most common cancers in men, followed by colorectal, stomach, and liver cancers. In terms of mortality in men, lung cancer has the highest rates followed by liver and stomach cancers. Breast cancer is by far the most common cancer diagnosed in women, followed by colorectal, cervix, and lung cancer.

In women, breast cancer is the most commonly occurring cancer in 140 countries of the world, while cervical cancer is the most common in 39 countries. Some countries have other cancer types as the most common in women, notably lung cancer in China, liver cancer in Mongolia, and thyroid cancer in South Korea. In men, prostate cancer is the most commonly diagnosed cancer in 87 countries worldwide, including all those in the Americas and in much of Europe, Australia, and parts of Africa. Lung cancer is the most common cancer in Russia, China, Eastern Europe, and parts of Northern Africa (38 countries). In Africa and Asia, there is more diversity in the most common sites in men.

③ Unlike the map for the most commonly diagnosed cancers, the global distribution of years of life lost to cancer shows much less variation and no relationship to level of development. This is because in many countries in Sub-Saharan Africa and Asia, a much higher proportion of fatal cancers are diagnosed at young ages.

②
Lung cancer is the leading cause of new cases and deaths among men, while breast cancer is the leading cause of new cases and deaths among women.

GLOBAL ESTIMATED AGE-STANDARDIZED CANCER INCIDENCE AND MORTALITY RATES (WORLD) PER 100,000 POPULATION, BY MAJOR SITES IN MEN AND WOMEN, 2012

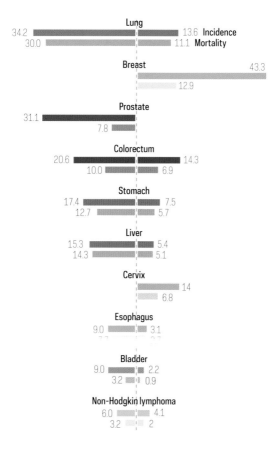

①
India, China, and other East and Central Asian countries account for nearly half of the world's new cancer cases and deaths.

ESTIMATED GLOBAL NUMBERS OF NEW CASES AND DEATHS BY MAJOR WORLD REGIONS, FOR ALL MALIGNANT CANCERS (EXCLUDING NON-MELANOMA SKIN CANCER) IN BOTH SEXES COMBINED, 2012

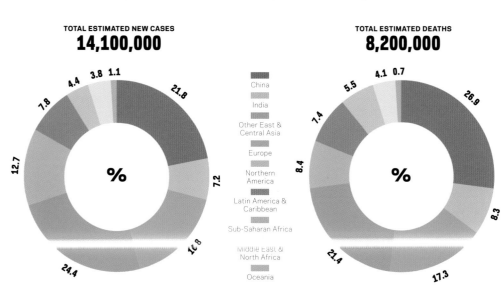

TOTAL ESTIMATED NEW CASES
14,100,000

TOTAL ESTIMATED DEATHS
8,200,000

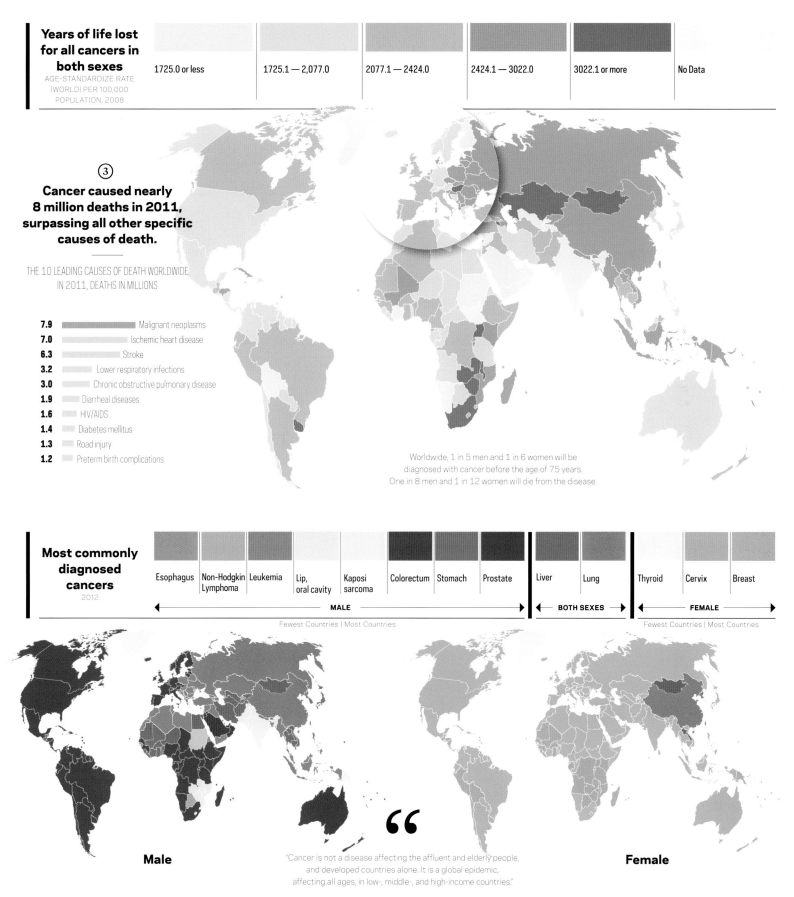

Years of life lost for all cancers in both sexes

AGE-STANDARDIZE RATE (WORLD) PER 100,000 POPULATION, 2008

| 1725.0 or less | 1725.1 — 2,077.0 | 2077.1 — 2424.0 | 2424.1 — 3022.0 | 3022.1 or more | No Data |

③

Cancer caused nearly 8 million deaths in 2011, surpassing all other specific causes of death.

THE 10 LEADING CAUSES OF DEATH WORLDWIDE IN 2011, DEATHS IN MILLIONS

7.9	Malignant neoplasms
7.0	Ischemic heart disease
6.3	Stroke
3.2	Lower respiratory infections
3.0	Chronic obstructive pulmonary disease
1.9	Diarrheal diseases
1.6	HIV/AIDS
1.4	Diabetes mellitus
1.3	Road injury
1.2	Preterm birth complications

Worldwide, 1 in 5 men and 1 in 6 women will be diagnosed with cancer before the age of 75 years. One in 8 men and 1 in 12 women will die from the disease.

Most commonly diagnosed cancers

2012

Esophagus | Non-Hodgkin Lymphoma | Leukemia | Lip, oral cavity | Kaposi sarcoma | Colorectum | Stomach | Prostate

← MALE →

Liver | Lung

← BOTH SEXES →

Thyroid | Cervix | Breast

← FEMALE →

Fewest Countries | Most Countries

Fewest Countries | Most Countries

Male

Female

❝

"Cancer is not a disease affecting the affluent and elderly people, and developed countries alone. It is a global epidemic, affecting all ages, in low-, middle-, and high-income countries."

— *Dr. Luis Gomes Sambo, Director of the WHO Regional Office for Africa, 2014*

LUNG CANCER

For several decades, lung cancer has been the most common cancer diagnosed and the leading cause of death from cancer in the world.

---

① There were an estimated 1.8 million new cases of lung cancer diagnosed in 2012 (13% of all new cancer cases), 58% of which occurred in less-developed regions. It is the most common cancer in men worldwide (1.2 million, 16.7% of all cases), with the highest estimated age-standardized incidence rates in Central and Eastern Europe (53.5 per 100,000) and Eastern Asia (50.4 per 100,000). Notably low incidence rates are observed in Middle and Western Africa (2.0 and 1.7 per 100,000, respectively). In women, the incidence rates are generally lower and the geographical pattern is a little different, reflecting varied historical patterns of tobacco use. Thus, the highest estimated rates are in Northern America (33.8) and Northern Europe (23.7), with a relatively high rate in Eastern Asia (19.2), and the lowest rates again in Western and Middle Africa (1.1 and 0.8 respectively).

Lung cancer is responsible for nearly one in five cancer deaths worldwide (1.6 million deaths, 19.4% of all cancer deaths) and is the leading cause of cancer death in men in 87 countries and in women in 26 countries. Because of its high fatality (the overall ratio of mortality to incidence is 0.87) and the relative lack of variability in survival in different world regions, the geographical patterns in mortality closely follow those in incidence, irrespective of level of resources in a given country.

② Recent trends in lung cancer reflect historical patterns of tobacco smoking.
③ In men, incidence rates have peaked and are now falling in several highly-developed countries, consistent with the initial adoption and subsequent decline in smoking some decades earlier. In most of these same countries, rates continue to rise among women as there has been no decline in smoking similar to that in men. However, in a few countries where smoking prevalence in women has been declining for several decades (notably in the USA), there are recent downward incidence trends.

Much of the burden could be prevented through tobacco control. Tobacco control policies (including increasing tobacco taxes and implementing smoke-free laws) are key to the prevention of lung cancer (see chapter 26 — *Tobacco Control*).

---

①

Because survival from lung cancer varies little by region, global patterns of lung cancer mortality mirror those of incidence.

ESTIMATED NEW LUNG CANCER CASES AND PERCENTAGE OF NEW CASES BY REGION, 2012

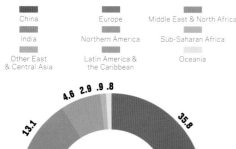

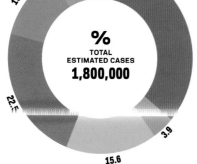

More than one third of all newly diagnosed cases of lung cancer occur in China.

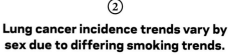

Lung cancer incidence trends vary by sex due to differing smoking trends.

AGE-STANDARDIZED INCIDENCE RATES (WORLD) PER 100,000 FOR SELECT COUNTRIES, BY SEX 1975-2011

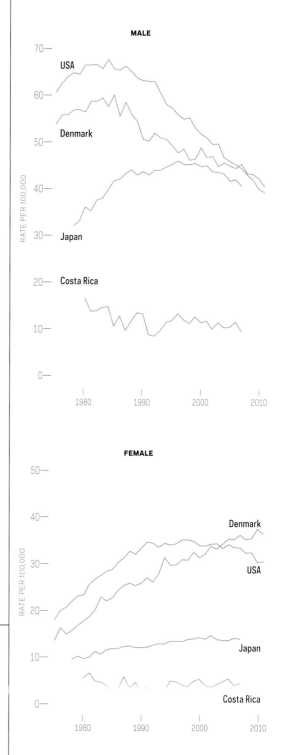

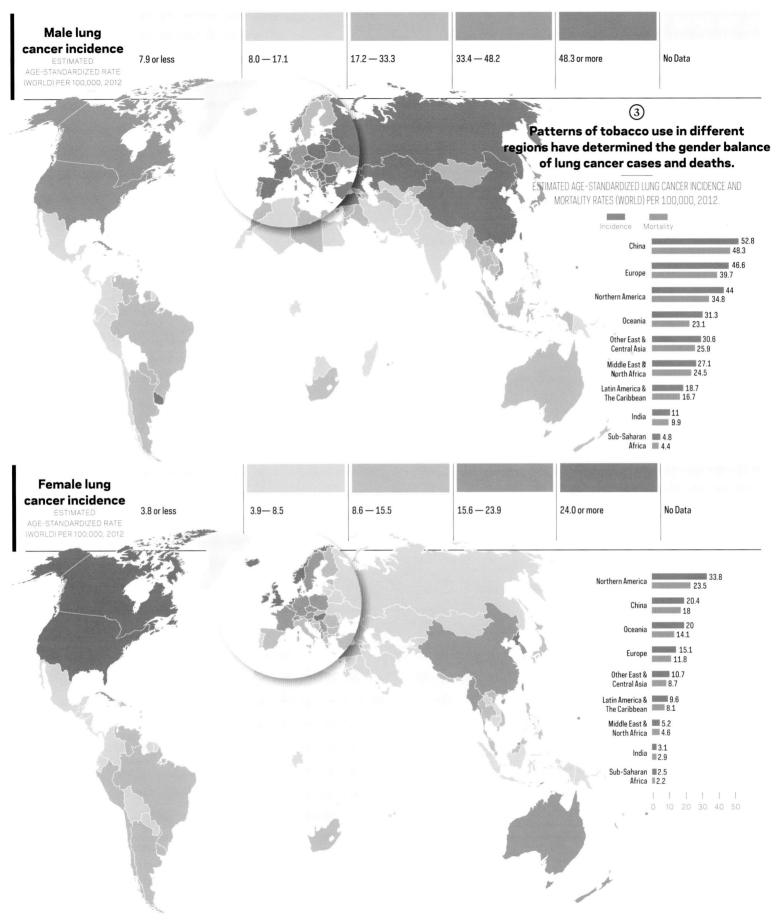

Male lung cancer incidence

ESTIMATED AGE-STANDARDIZED RATE (WORLD) PER 100,000, 2012

| 7.9 or less | 8.0 — 17.1 | 17.2 — 33.3 | 33.4 — 48.2 | 48.3 or more | No Data |

③

Patterns of tobacco use in different regions have determined the gender balance of lung cancer cases and deaths.

ESTIMATED AGE-STANDARDIZED LUNG CANCER INCIDENCE AND MORTALITY RATES (WORLD) PER 100,000, 2012.

Incidence   Mortality

Region	Incidence	Mortality
China	52.8	48.3
Europe	46.6	39.7
Northern America	44	34.8
Oceania	31.3	23.1
Other East & Central Asia	30.6	25.9
Middle East & North Africa	27.1	24.5
Latin America & The Caribbean	18.7	16.7
India	11	9.9
Sub-Saharan Africa	4.8	4.4

Female lung cancer incidence

ESTIMATED AGE-STANDARDIZED RATE (WORLD) PER 100,000, 2012

| 3.8 or less | 3.9 — 8.5 | 8.6 — 15.5 | 15.6 — 23.9 | 24.0 or more | No Data |

Region	Incidence	Mortality
Northern America	33.8	23.5
China	20.4	18
Oceania	20	14.1
Europe	15.1	11.8
Other East & Central Asia	10.7	8.7
Latin America & The Caribbean	9.6	8.1
Middle East & North Africa	5.2	4.6
India	3.1	2.9
Sub-Saharan Africa	2.5	2.2

0   10   20   30   40   50

BREAST CANCER

Breast cancer is by far the most frequently diagnosed cancer and cause of cancer death among women worldwide.

① Breast cancer is the most common cancer in women worldwide, with slightly more cases estimated in 2012 in less-developed (883,000 cases) than in more-developed (794,000) regions. Of the 184 countries included in the GLOBOCAN database, breast cancer is the most common cancer diagnosis in women in 140 countries (76%) and the most frequent cause of cancer mortality in 101 countries (55%).

③ Incidence rates vary nearly fourfold across the world regions, ranging from 27 per 100,000 in Middle Africa and Eastern Asia to 96 per 100,000 in Western Europe, and tend to be elevated in countries with highest development. Breast cancer is the most frequent cause of cancer death in women in less-developed regions (324,000 deaths, 14.3% of total) and the second cause of cancer death in more-developed regions (198,000 deaths, 15.4%), after lung cancer.

② Incidence rates continue to increase in all countries except in a few high-income countries. In contrast, mortality rates are decreasing in many high-income countries but increasing in low- and middle-income countries.

The variation in mortality rates between world regions (ranging from 6 per 100,000 in Eastern Asia to 20 per 100,000 in Western Africa) is less than that for incidence rates because of the considerably better survival from breast cancer in developed regions, resulting from increased access to early detection (mammography) and treatment. Differences in incidence between countries with and without mammography screening programs are also influenced by earlier diagnosis and the overdiagnosis associated with detecting breast cancers in asymptomatic women. Overall, a substantially greater proportion of women with breast cancer will die from their disease in less-developed regions.

---

② **Breast cancer incidence rates continue to increase in all countries except a few high-income countries, while mortality rates are decreasing in many high-income countries and increasing in low- and middle-income countries.**

AGE-STANDARDIZED INCIDENCE AND MORTALITY RATES (WORLD) PER 100,000 FOR SELECT COUNTRIES, 1975-2011

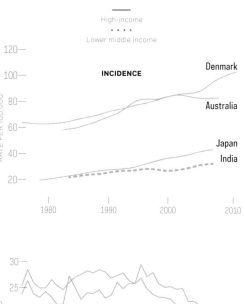

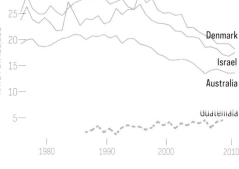

---

① **Although the estimated number of breast cancer deaths is less than a third of estimated new cases, breast cancer is the most common cause of cancer death in women in less-developed countries, and the second among women in developed countries.**

ESTIMATED NEW BREAST CANCER CASES AND DEATHS BY REGION, 2012

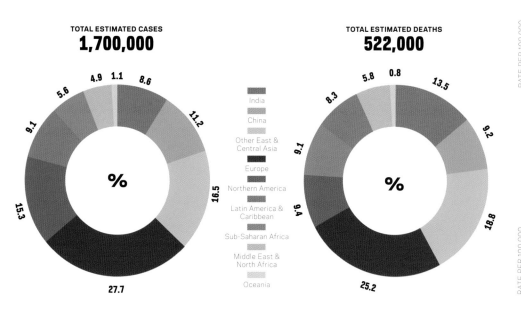

There were an estimated 1.7 million new cases (25% of all cancers in women) and 0.5 million cancer deaths (15% of all cancer deaths in women) in 2012.

Female Breast Cancer Incidence

ESTIMATED AGE-STANDARDIZED RATE (WORLD) PER 100,000 POPULATION, 2012

| 26.0 or less | 26.01—39.6 | 39.7 — 55.8 | 55.8 — 76.2 | 76.3 or more | No Data |

③

Although incidence rates are highest in developed regions, mortality rates in these areas are comparable to most of the less-developed regions.

ESTIMATED AGE-STANDARDIZED FEMALE BREAST CANCER INCIDENCE RATE (WORLD) PER 100,000, 2012

- 91.6 Northern America
- 79.2 Oceania
- 71.1 Europe
- 47.2 Latin America & the Caribbean
- 43.0 Middle East & North Africa
- 38.3 East & Central Asia
- 33.8 Sub-Saharan Africa
- 25.8 India
- 22.1 China

Female Breast Cancer Mortality

ESTIMATED AGE-STANDARDIZED RATE (WORLD) PER 100,000 POPULATION, 2012

| 8.1 or less | 8.2—12.0 | 12.1 — 15.9 | 16.0 — 20.7 | 20.8 or more | No Data |

ESTIMATED AGE-STANDARDIZED FEMALE BREAST CANCER MORTALITY RATE (WORLD) PER 100,000, 2012

- 17.2 Sub-Saharan Africa
- 16.2 Middle East & North Africa
- 16.1 Europe
- 15.6 Oceania
- 14.8 Northern America
- 13.7 East & Central Asia
- 13 Latin America & the Caribbean
- 12.7 India
- 5.4 China

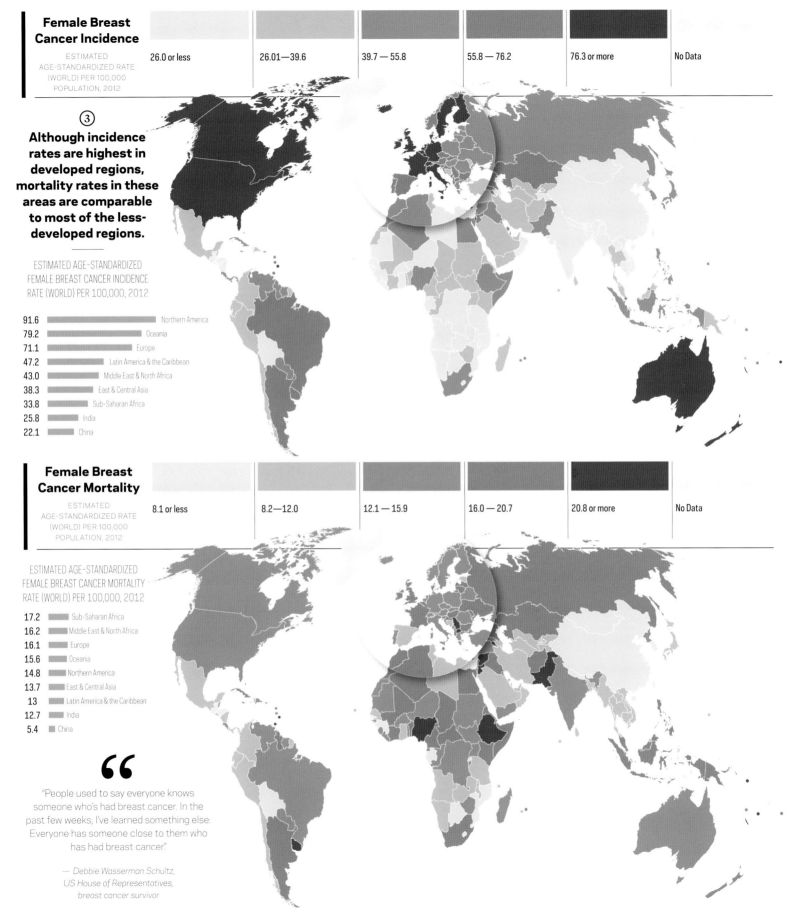

"People used to say everyone knows someone who's had breast cancer. In the past few weeks, I've learned something else: Everyone has someone close to them who has had breast cancer."

— Debbie Wasserman Schultz,
US House of Representatives,
breast cancer survivor

CANCER IN CHILDREN

Survival among children with cancer is improving, but children in low-income countries continue to have worse outcomes than those in high-income countries.

①② Childhood cancers account for less than 1% of the total cases in high-income countries but about 4% in low-income countries. The types of cancers that occur in children differ from those of adults and mainly comprise neoplasms of the blood and lymphatic system (leukemia or lymphoma), embryonal tumors (e.g. retinoblastoma, neuroblastoma, nephroblastoma) and tumors of brain, bones, and connective tissues, with international variations. Overall estimated annual incidence rates vary between 50 and 200 per million in children under 15 years of age, and between 90 and 300 per million in adolescents aged 15–19. Reliable data on incidence are available for a fifth of the world population, mostly in high-income countries.

Established causes of childhood cancers include ionizing radiation, genetic constitution and viruses, while suspected risk factors include birth characteristics and exposure to certain pollutants.

③ While fifty years ago only about 30% of childhood cancer patients survived five years following diagnosis, the current proportion is now 80% in high-income countries but remain low in low- and middle-income countries (e.g. 40% in India). ④ Survival data for low-income countries are sparse, but the annual estimated number of deaths exceeds half of new cases in Africa, Asia and Latin America. National investments and international collaboration could improve these outcomes.

As survival improves, the population of long-term survivors grows. In 2012 in the USA alone, there were 80,000 survivors diagnosed with cancer before the age of 20 years. About 60% of survivors suffer at least one chronic condition, and the risk of late effects increases with length of follow-up. New therapies should overcome the recent slowdown in survival improvement and reduce the late effects of treatment.

①
The proportion of childhood cancers relative to all cancers is highest in low-Human Development Index (HDI) countries with young populations.

CANCER IN CHILDREN (AGE 0–14 YEARS)
AS A PERCENTAGE OF CANCERS IN ALL AGES

Cases
Deaths

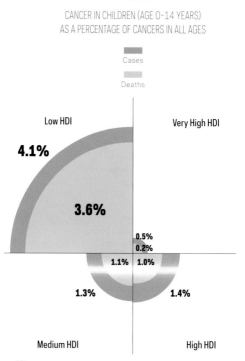

Low HDI
Very High HDI
4.1%
3.6%
0.5%
0.2%
1.1% 1.0%
1.3% 1.4%
Medium HDI
High HDI

④
The ratio of childhood cancer incidence to mortality is lower in low-HDI countries.

ESTIMATED RATES PER MILLION OF CANCER INCIDENCE AND MORTALITY IN CHILDREN (AGE 0–14 YEARS), 2012

Incidence

Mortality

HIGHEST HDI REGIONS ← → LOWEST HDI REGIONS

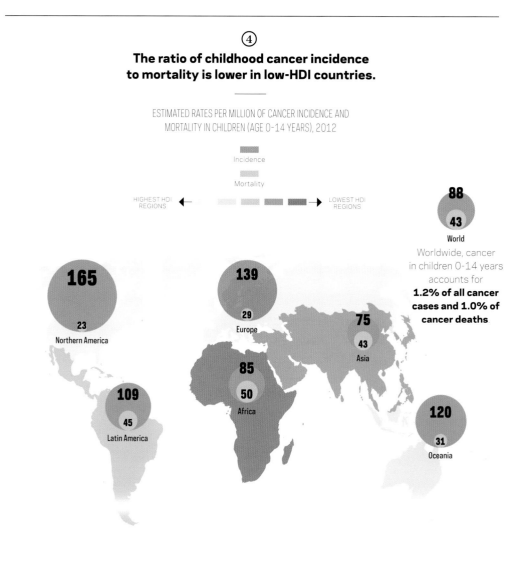

88
43
World
Worldwide, cancer in children 0–14 years accounts for **1.2% of all cancer cases and 1.0% of cancer deaths**

165
23
Northern America

139
29
Europe

75
43
Asia

85
50
Africa

109
45
Latin America

120
31
Oceania

Cancers in children are mostly neoplasms of the blood and lymphatic system (leukemia or lymphoma), embryonal tumors (e.g. retinoblastoma, neuroblastoma, nephroblastoma) and tumors of brain, bones, and connective tissues.

VARIATION IN AGE-STANDARDIZED CHILDHOOD CANCER INCIDENCE RATES (WORLD), PER MILLION POPULATION

1 new case per million population

	Australia 1997-2006	USA 2002-2010	France 2000-2004	Argentina 2000-2008	Iran 2004-2006	China, Shanghai 2002-2005	Thailand 2003-2005	India, Chennai 2002-2005	Uganda, Kyadondo 1993-1997	Zimbabwe, Harare 1990-1997
Leukemia										
Lymphoma										
Nervous System Tumors (CNS and Neuroblastoma)										
Retinoblastoma										
Wilms & Other Renal Tumors										
Kaposi Sarcoma										
Bone & Other Soft Tissue Sarcomas										
Germ Cell Tumors										
Epithelial Neoplasms and Melanoma										
Other & Unspecified										

HIGHEST HDI ◄———————————————————► LOWEST HDI

Survival from childhood cancer varies internationally.

FIVE-YEAR SURVIVAL IN CHILDREN FOR SELECT CANCERS DIAGNOSED IN SELECT COUNTRIES

Survival %

	Australia, 1997-2006	China, Shanghai, 2002-2005	Thailand, 2003-2005	India, Chennai, 2002-2005
Leukemia	80.6%	52.2%	57.4%	36.3%
Lymphoma	89.9%	58.8%	59.5%	55.3%
Nervous System Tumors	71.0%	41.2%	41.7%	26.8%
All Cancers	79.6%	55.7%	54.9%	40.0%
	1997-2006	2002-2005	2003-2004	1990-2001

HIGHEST HDI ◄————————————► LOWEST HDI

Over half of children with cancer have **leukemia, lymphoma, or brain tumors.**

"

"There are no great discoveries and advances, as long as there is an unhappy child on earth."

— *Albert Einstein*

In the USA, childhood cancer survival has significantly improved over the past 30 years, although racial disparities remain.

PERCENTAGE OF PATIENTS (AGE 0-19 YEARS) SURVIVING 5 YEARS AFTER THEIR CANCER DIAGNOSIS IN THE USA

White

Black

90% — 80% — 70% — 60% — 50% —

1975   1980   1985   1990   1995   2000   2005

YEARS OF DIAGNOSIS

HUMAN DEVELOPMENT INDEX (HDI) TRANSITIONS

HDI transitions lead to changes in the scale and profile of cancer occurrence.

①

As countries transition towards higher levels of human development, their cancer burden will not only increase, but the types of cancer observed will also change.

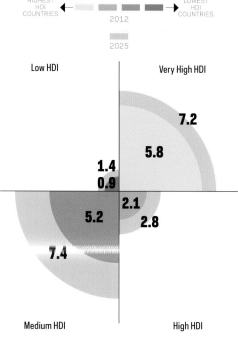

RECENT (2012) AND FUTURE (2025) CANCER BURDEN BY HDI (NEW CASES IN MILLIONS), BASED ON PROJECTED DEMOGRAPHIC CHANGES

HIGHEST HDI COUNTRIES ← 2012 → LOWEST HDI COUNTRIES

2025

Low HDI | Very High HDI

7.2
5.8
1.4
0.9
2.1
5.2
2.8
7.4

Medium HDI | High HDI

① Changes in fertility and life expectancy are leading to a rapidly growing and aging world population—and an unsurpassed scale of the cancer problem—as countries undergo major transitions in development. As such, the traditional grouping of regions of the world into "more-developed" and "less-developed" is less relevant today. The Human Development Index (HDI), a composite measure of educational attainment and life expectancy, as well as level of income, is the best contemporary measure for socioeconomic development of countries.

Cancers of the colorectum, lung, female breast, prostate, and stomach were the most commonly diagnosed cancers in both very high-HDI and high-HDI areas in 2012. Lung cancer is the most common neoplasm in medium-HDI areas. In the low-HDI areas, comprising mainly countries in Sub-Saharan Africa, the cancer profile is quite different, with cervical and female breast cancer ranked as the first and second most common cancers in both sexes combined in 2012, and with a number of predominantly infection-related cancers still very common.

② The evolution of cancers in women shows a consistent and very striking pattern that includes rapid declines in the incidence of cervical cancer offset by concurrent increases in female breast cancer. The earlier the year in which the two cancers intersect is a marker of the extent of economic transition in a given country.

③ By 2025, 19 million new cancer cases will be diagnosed in men and women based solely on projected demographic changes. The increases in cancer incidence are proportionally greatest in lower-HDI settings.

②

The year of intersection of rates following secular declines in cervical cancer and rises in breast cancer is generally a marker of degree of socioeconomic transition.

TRENDS IN FEMALE BREAST VS. CERVICAL CANCER INCIDENCE 1975-2010 IN SELECT COUNTRIES BY HDI STATUS.

Breast Cancer
Cervical Cancer

RATES PER 100,000

100 —
80 —
60 —
40 —
20 —
0 —

Denmark 1975 – 2010 | Colombia 1983 – 2007 | India 1983 – 2007 | Uganda 1993 – 2007

HIGHEST HDI ← → LOWEST HDI

Human Development Index Ranking

UNITED NATIONS DEVELOPMENT PROGRAMME, 2013

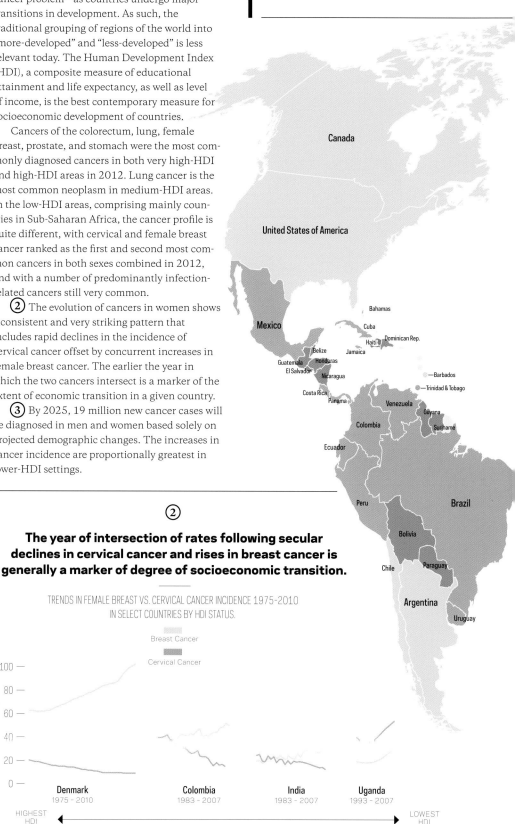

Canada
United States of America
Mexico
Bahamas
Cuba
Haiti
Dominican Rep.
Belize
Jamaica
Guatemala
Honduras
El Salvador
Nicaragua
Barbados
Trinidad & Tobago
Costa Rica
Panama
Venezuela
Guyana
Colombia
Suriname
Ecuador
Peru
Brazil
Bolivia
Chile
Paraguay
Argentina
Uruguay

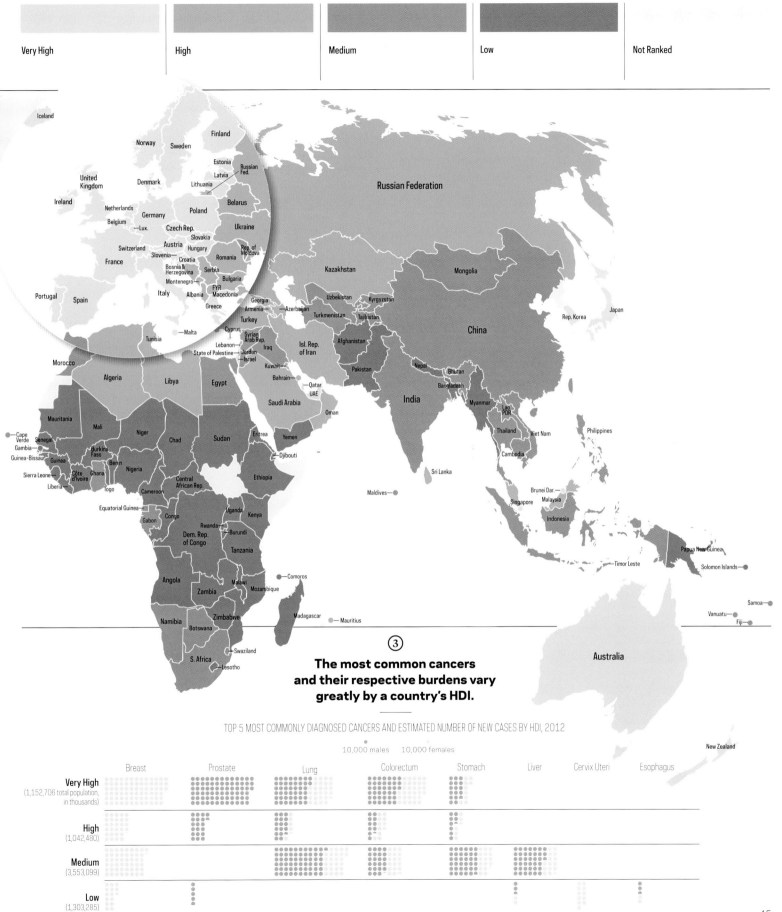

③

The most common cancers and their respective burdens vary greatly by a country's HDI.

TOP 5 MOST COMMONLY DIAGNOSED CANCERS AND ESTIMATED NUMBER OF NEW CASES BY HDI, 2012

10,000 males   10,000 females

	Breast	Prostate	Lung	Colorectum	Stomach	Liver	Cervix Uteri	Esophagus
Very High (1,152,706 total population, in thousands)								
High (1,042,480)								
Medium (3,553,099)								
Low (1,303,285)								

OVERVIEW OF GEOGRAPHICAL DIVERSITY

The cancer incidence and mortality profile of a given country or region is the product of a mix of risk factors, screening and early detection efforts, and access to adequate treatment.

Across the globe there are striking geographical differences in cancer occurrence, mortality and survival. ① The relatively high rates of liver, stomach, and cervical cancer in some countries in Asia, South America, and Sub-Saharan Africa are partly due to the high prevalence of chronic infection of hepatitis, *Helicobacter pylori* and human papillomavirus (HPV), respectively. In Sub-Saharan Africa, there is a staggeringly high rate of Kaposi sarcoma due to the high prevalence of HIV infection. ② In contrast, rates of infection-related cancers are very low in Europe and North America, where cancers linked to lifestyle "westernization" such as colorectal and breast dominate the regional profile. These populations are further distinguished by their large burden of prostate and lung cancer, as well as the notably high rate of skin melanoma.

③ The variation in the occurrence of cancer types between different parts of the world gives some indication of the proportion of cancers that could be prevented by modifying specific harmful lifestyle or environmental factors. Removal of HPV infection would substantially reduce the burden of cervical cancer; smoking and indoor and outdoor air pollution explain over two-thirds of lung cancer incidence. ④ Yet, for many cancers, the causes remain largely unknown. Only 5–20% of all prostate, colorectal and breast cancers could be prevented by better diet, increased physical activity, or reduced alcohol consumption.

In addition to differences in risk factors, higher awareness in the population combined with more widespread early detection practices also explain the national and regional variation for some cancers.

Finally, regional differences in incidence will be reflected in mortality. Yet death from cancer is also influenced by early detection and access to adequate treatment. ⑤ For example, less access to diagnosis and treatment facilities for prostate cancer is partly responsible for the higher mortality observed in low-income settings. On the other hand, for cancers for which treatment does not greatly affect survival, e.g. liver cancer, the regional mortality profile mimics that of incidence.

①

Liver and cervical cancers are more common in regions where infection-related causes are more prevalent.

ESTIMATED INCIDENCE OF LIVER CANCER (AGE-STANDARDIZED RATE [WORLD] PER 100,000) IN MALES IN 2012

| 6.8 or less | 6.9–13.8 | 13.9–25.8 | 25.9–40.2 | 40.3 or more | No Data |

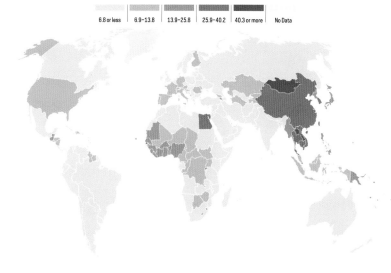

ESTIMATED INCIDENCE OF CERVICAL CANCER (AGE-STANDARDIZED RATE [WORLD] PER 100,000) IN FEMALES IN 2012

| 10.0 or less | 10.1–18.0 | 18.1–27.6 | 27.7–41.8 | 41.9 or more | No Data |

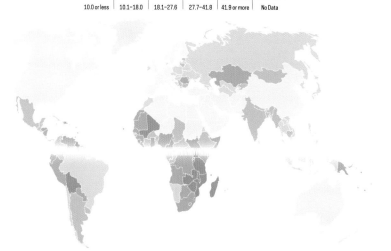

③

Variations in incidence rates of some cancers largely reflect differences in distribution of risk factors.

HIGHEST AND LOWEST INCIDENCE RATES (AGE-STANDARDIZED RATE [WORLD] PER 100,000) BY CANCER SITE AND SEX, 2003–2007

Example cancer registries with markedly high and low rates are labeled

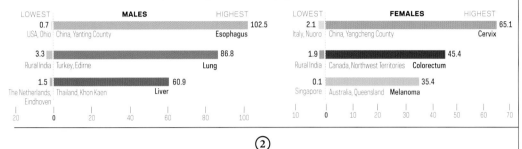

LOWEST	**MALES**	HIGHEST		LOWEST	**FEMALES**	HIGHEST
0.7 USA, Ohio	China, Yanting County	102.5 Esophagus		2.1 Italy, Nuoro	China, Yangcheng County	65.1 Cervix
3.3 Rural India	Turkey, Edirne	86.8 Lung		1.9 Rural India	Canada, Northwest Territories	45.4 Colorectum
1.5 The Netherlands, Eindhoven	Thailand, Khon Kaen	60.9 Liver		0.1 Singapore	Australia, Queensland	35.4 Melanoma

②

Colorectal cancer dominates in "westernized" cultures.

ESTIMATED INCIDENCE OF COLORECTAL CANCER (AGE-STANDARDIZED RATE [WORLD] PER 100,000) IN BOTH SEXES IN 2012

6.1 or less | 6.2–12.1 | 12.2–20.5 | 20.6–30.2 | 30.3 or more | No Data

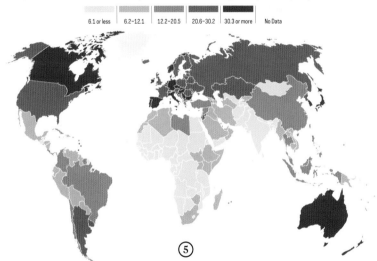

⑤

Higher mortality from prostate cancer generally reflects lower access to diagnosis and treatment facilities.

ESTIMATED MORTALITY FROM PROSTATE CANCER (AGE-STANDARDIZED RATE [WORLD] PER 100,000) IN MALES IN 2012

7.4 or less | 7.5–14.2 | 14.3–22.8 | 22.9–36.6 | 36.7 or more | No Data

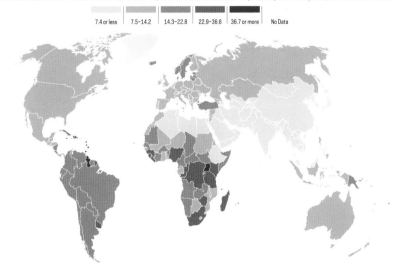

④

The causes of a large portion of commonly diagnosed cancers in Western populations remains unknown.

ESTIMATED NUMBER OF NEW CANCER CASES (2012) AND PERCENT ATTRIBUTABLE TO UNKNOWN RISK FACTORS BY CANCER SITE

Unknown causes

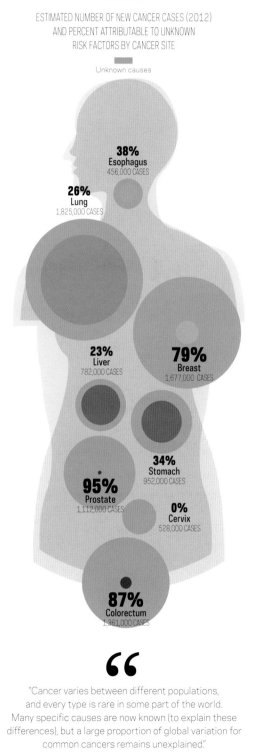

38% Esophagus 456,000 CASES

26% Lung 1,825,000 CASES

23% Liver 782,000 CASES

79% Breast 1,677,000 CASES

95% Prostate 1,112,000 CASES

34% Stomach 952,000 CASES

0% Cervix 528,000 CASES

87% Colorectum 1,361,000 CASES

"

"Cancer varies between different populations, and every type is rare in some part of the world. Many specific causes are now known (to explain these differences), but a large proportion of global variation for common cancers remains unexplained."

— Peto J. *Nature*, 2001.

REGIONAL DIVERSITY

Cancer in Sub-Saharan Africa

In Sub-Saharan Africa, infection-related cancers are still common, although cancers associated with social and economic transition are becoming increasingly frequent.

Cancer is emerging as a major public health problem in Sub-Saharan Africa (SSA) because of population aging and growth, as well as increased prevalence of key risk factors, including those associated with social and economic transition. A high residual burden of infectious agents (HIV/AIDS, human papillomavirus, hepatitis B virus) in certain SSA countries still drives the rates of certain cancers; about one-third of all cancers in the region are estimated to be infection-related.

(1) In females, the numbers of cases and rates of breast and cervical cancer are almost equal and comprise 50% of the overall cancer burden in SSA. In males, cancer of the prostate dominates in terms of the number of cases (51,900 cases, 27.9% of the total estimated cases in the region), followed by liver cancer (10.6% of the total) and Kaposi sarcoma (6.6% of the total).

(2) Breast and cervical cancer in women and prostate cancer in men are the major cancers that define the overall risk of developing and dying from cancer in SSA. Around one in 26 women will develop cervical cancer in their lifetime, and one in 40 will die from the disease. The lifetime risks for women developing breast cancer and men developing prostate cancer are very similar to those for women developing cervical cancer, but the lifetime risk of dying from either of these two cancers (approximately one in 55) is slightly less.

There are, however, large variations in the cancer profile in different countries, with prostate cancer dominating in men (most frequent in 23 countries), and cervical or breast cancer the most frequent in women in 28 and 19 countries respectively. In men, there are a number of countries where liver and Kaposi sarcoma are the most common cancers, in Western and Eastern regions of Africa, respectively.

(3) Cancer control action in SSA will require measures that address the persistently high incidence of cancers associated with poverty and infection (including a residual burden of AIDS-associated cancers), in addition to emerging cancers associated with economic development.

---

(2)

For many cancers, the risk of getting cancer and the risk of dying from it are nearly the same in Sub-Saharan Africa, because of late stage at diagnosis and lack of treatment.

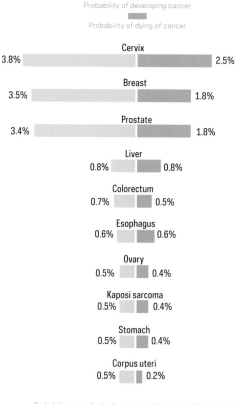

PROBABILITY OF DEVELOPING OR DYING FROM CANCER BEFORE THE AGE OF 75 IN SUB-SAHARAN AFRICA, 2012

Probability of developing cancer
Probability of dying of cancer

	Developing	Dying
Cervix	3.8%	2.5%
Breast	3.5%	1.8%
Prostate	3.4%	1.8%
Liver	0.8%	0.8%
Colorectum	0.7%	0.5%
Esophagus	0.6%	0.6%
Ovary	0.5%	0.4%
Kaposi sarcoma	0.5%	0.4%
Stomach	0.5%	0.4%
Corpus uteri	0.5%	0.2%

Probabilities are for both sexes combined, with the exception of cervical, breast, and prostate cancers.

"

"We cannot afford to say, 'We must tackle other diseases first— HIV/AIDS, malaria, tuberculosis—then we will deal with chronic diseases.' If we wait even 10 years, we will find that the problem is even larger and more expensive to address."

— *Olusegun Obasanjo, former President of Nigeria*

---

(1)

Breast, cervix, prostate and liver cancers, along with Kaposi sarcoma, predominate in Sub-Saharan Africa, both in cases and in deaths.

ESTIMATED NUMBERS OF NEW CANCER CASES AND DEATHS, BOTH SEXES, 2012

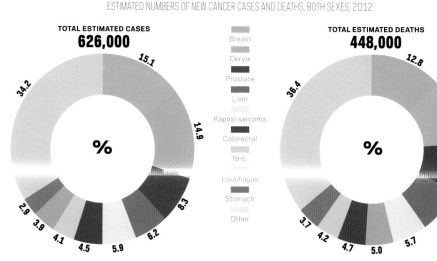

TOTAL ESTIMATED CASES
626,000

34.2 / 15.1 / 14.9 / 8.3 / 6.2 / 5.9 / 4.5 / 4.1 / 3.9 / 2.9

Breast
Cervix
Prostate
Liver
Kaposi sarcoma
Colorectal
NHL
Esophagus
Stomach
Other

TOTAL ESTIMATED DEATHS
448,000

36.4 / 12.8 / 10.6 / 8.3 / 5.7 / 5.0 / 4.7 / 4.2 / 3.7

Most commonly diagnosed cancers
2012

Stomach	Esophagus	Non-Hodgkin lymphoma	Leukemia	Colorectum	Kaposi sarcoma	Liver	Prostate

◄——————————————— MALE ———————————————►

Breast	Cervix

◄—— FEMALE ——►

Fewest Countries | Most Countries   Fewest Countries | Most Countries

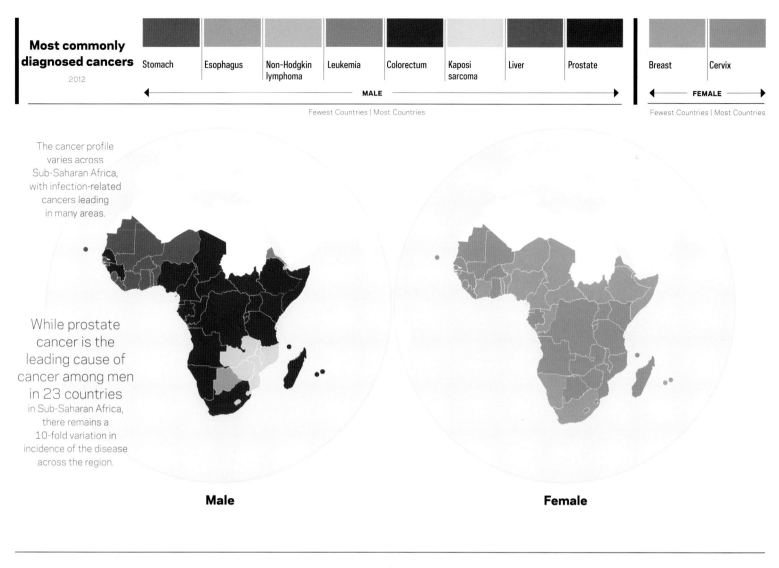

The cancer profile varies across Sub-Saharan Africa, with infection-related cancers leading in many areas.

While prostate cancer is the leading cause of cancer among men in 23 countries in Sub-Saharan Africa, there remains a 10-fold variation in incidence of the disease across the region.

Male

Female

③

**Kaposi sarcoma incidence rates have been declining since the late 1990's in Zimbabwe, reflective of the waning HIV/AIDS epidemic in this country.
In contrast, incidence rates for prostate, breast, and cervical cancers have steadily increased over the past 20 years.**

AVERAGE ANNUAL AGE-STANDARDIZED INCIDENCE RATES (WORLD) FOR COMMON CANCERS AMONG THE BLACK POPULATION OF HARARE, 1991-2010.

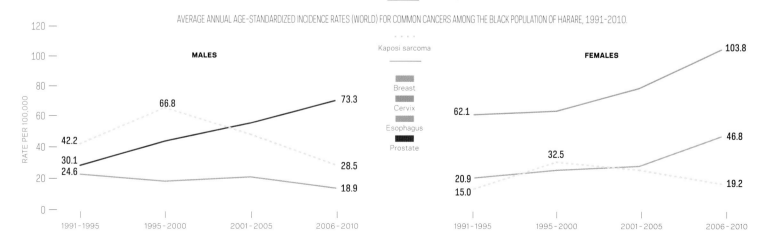

MALES

Kaposi sarcoma
Breast
Cervix
Esophagus
Prostate

FEMALES

RATE PER 100,000

120
100
80
60
40
20
0

Males: 66.8, 42.2, 30.1, 24.6, 73.3, 28.5, 18.9

Females: 62.1, 103.8, 46.8, 32.5, 20.9, 15.0, 19.2

1991-1995   1995-2000   2001-2005   2006-2010

REGIONAL DIVERSITY

Cancer in Latin America and the Caribbean

Prostate cancer is the leading cause of cancer death among males, while breast cancer is the leading cause among females. Lung cancer is also a major cause of cancer death among both sexes.

① About 1.1 million new cancer cases and 600,000 cancer deaths are estimated to occur annually in Latin America and the Caribbean. Prostate cancer is the leading cause of cancer death among males, with about 51,000 deaths annually, followed by lung cancer and stomach cancer. Among females, breast cancer is the leading cause of cancer death, with about 43,000 deaths annually, followed by cervical and lung cancer.

There is considerable variation in cancer rates and trends within Latin America. For example, cervical cancer incidence rates in 2012 ranged from 11.4 cases per 100,000 population in Costa Rica to 47.7 cases per 100,000 in Bolivia, with the highest rates generally found in low-income countries. ② Cervical cancer rates are decreasing in many countries due to increased screening, while breast cancer rates are increasing due to increased prevalence of hormonally-linked factors such as delayed childbearing and lower parity, as well as lifestyle risk factors. Gallbladder cancer rates are exceptionally high in many Latin American countries, especially Chile and Bolivia, for unknown reasons. ③ Lung cancer mortality rates have begun to stabilize or decrease among males in many middle-income countries of the Americas, such as Argentina and Brazil, because of decreased smoking prevalence. Notably, lung cancer mortality rates among females continue to increase in most countries of the Americas, reflecting the lag in smoking reduction.

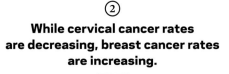

②

While cervical cancer rates are decreasing, breast cancer rates are increasing.

TRENDS IN CERVICAL AND FEMALE BREAST CANCER INCIDENCE, AGE-STANDARDIZED RATES* (WORLD) PER 100,000 POPULATION, ALL AGES, RATES PER 100,000, 1981-2006

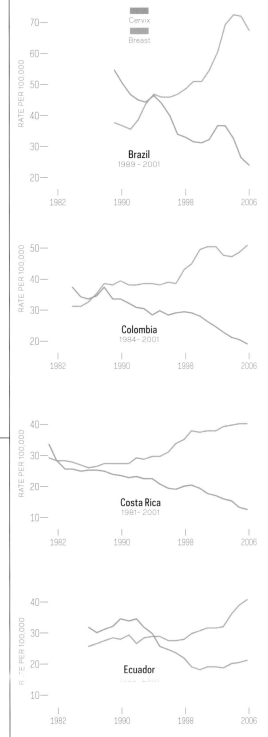

*Rates have been smoothed using 3-year averages

①

Lung cancer is the leading cause of cancer death for both sexes combined.

ESTIMATED NUMBERS OF NEW CANCER CASES AND DEATHS, BOTH SEXES, 2012

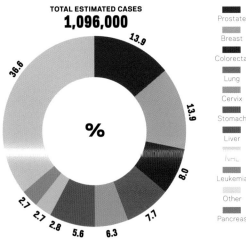

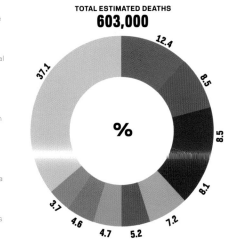

TOTAL ESTIMATED CASES
1,096,000

TOTAL ESTIMATED DEATHS
603,000

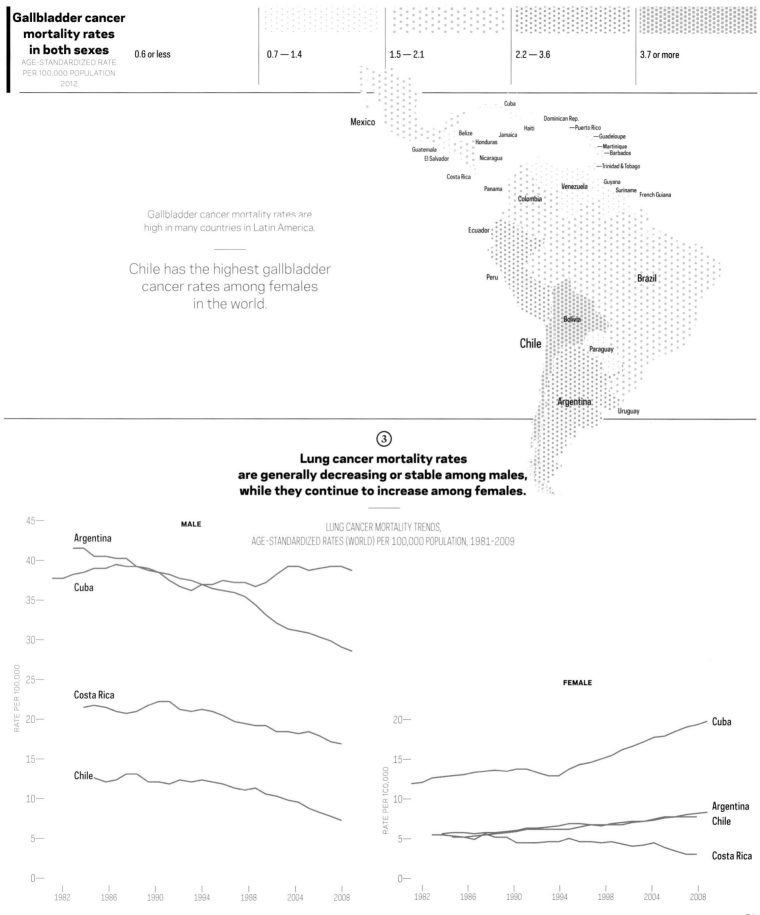

Gallbladder cancer mortality rates in both sexes

AGE-STANDARDIZED RATE PER 100,000 POPULATION 2012

| 0.6 or less | 0.7 — 1.4 | 1.5 — 2.1 | 2.2 — 3.6 | 3.7 or more |

Gallbladder cancer mortality rates are high in many countries in Latin America.

———

Chile has the highest gallbladder cancer rates among females in the world.

Mexico
Cuba
Belize
Guatemala
El Salvador
Honduras
Jamaica
Haiti
Dominican Rep.
—Puerto Rico
—Guadeloupe
—Martinique
—Barbados
—Trinidad & Tobago
Nicaragua
Costa Rica
Panama
Colombia
Venezuela
Guyana
Suriname
French Guiana
Ecuador
Peru
Brazil
Bolivia
Chile
Paraguay
Argentina
Uruguay

③

Lung cancer mortality rates are generally decreasing or stable among males, while they continue to increase among females.

———

LUNG CANCER MORTALITY TRENDS, AGE-STANDARDIZED RATES (WORLD) PER 100,000 POPULATION, 1981-2009

MALE

Argentina
Cuba
Costa Rica
Chile

RATE PER 100,000

45—
40—
35—
30—
25—
20—
15—
10—
5—
0—

1982 1986 1990 1994 1998 2004 2008

FEMALE

Cuba
Argentina
Chile
Costa Rica

RATE PER 100,000

20—
15—
10—
5—
0—

1982 1986 1990 1994 1998 2004 2008

REGIONAL DIVERSITY

Cancer in Northern America

Not all segments of the Northern American population have benefited equally from scientific advances in cancer prevention and control.

About 1.79 million new cancer cases and 692,000 cancer deaths were estimated to have occurred in 2012 in Northern America. ① Prostate cancer in males and breast cancer in females are the most commonly diagnosed cancers, followed by lung and colorectal cancers in both males and females.

Rates and trends in incidence, mortality, and survival for all cancers combined and for most cancers are generally similar between the USA and Canada. ② For example, incidence rates have continued to increase for kidney and thyroid cancer, in part because of wide application of imaging techniques, and for liver cancer because of the high prevalence of hepatitis C virus infections during the 1970s and 1980s due to intravenous drug use. In contrast, rates have continued to decrease for lung and cervical cancer because of reduced cigarette smoking and increased use of Pap testing, respectively.

However, national cancer rates and trends mask marked differences between subpopulations, especially in the USA. For example, lung cancer rates are highest in Southern and Midwestern states, which have been historically dependent on tobacco farming and production. ③ ④ Progress in reducing colorectal and breast cancer mortality rates lags in blacks compared to whites, and survival after a diagnosis of cancer is lower in uninsured than in insured patients due to unequal access to medical care.

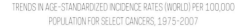

High prevalence of hepatitis C virus in the 1970s and 1980s in part accounts for the increase in liver cancer incidence, while reduced smoking and more Pap testing for the decrease in lung and cervical cancer rates, respectively.

TRENDS IN AGE-STANDARDIZED INCIDENCE RATES (WORLD) PER 100,000 POPULATION FOR SELECT CANCERS, 1975-2007

—— USA
····· Canada

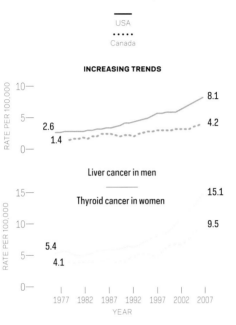

INCREASING TRENDS

Liver cancer in men

Thyroid cancer in women

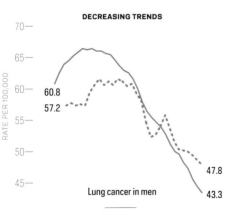

DECREASING TRENDS

Lung cancer in men

Cervical cancer in women

---

①

Prostate cancer in males and breast cancer in females are the most commonly diagnosed cancers, followed by lung and colorectal cancers in both sexes combined. Lung cancer is the leading cause of cancer death.

ESTIMATED NUMBERS OF NEW CANCER CASES AND DEATHS, BOTH SEXES, 2012

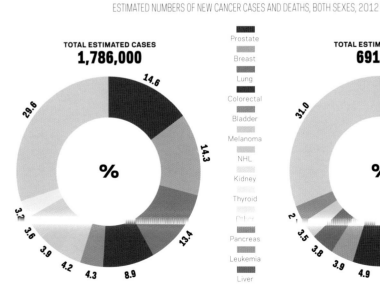

TOTAL ESTIMATED CASES
1,786,000

TOTAL ESTIMATED DEATHS
691,000

Prostate
Breast
Lung
Colorectal
Bladder
Melanoma
NHL
Kidney
Thyroid
Other
Pancreas
Leukemia
Liver

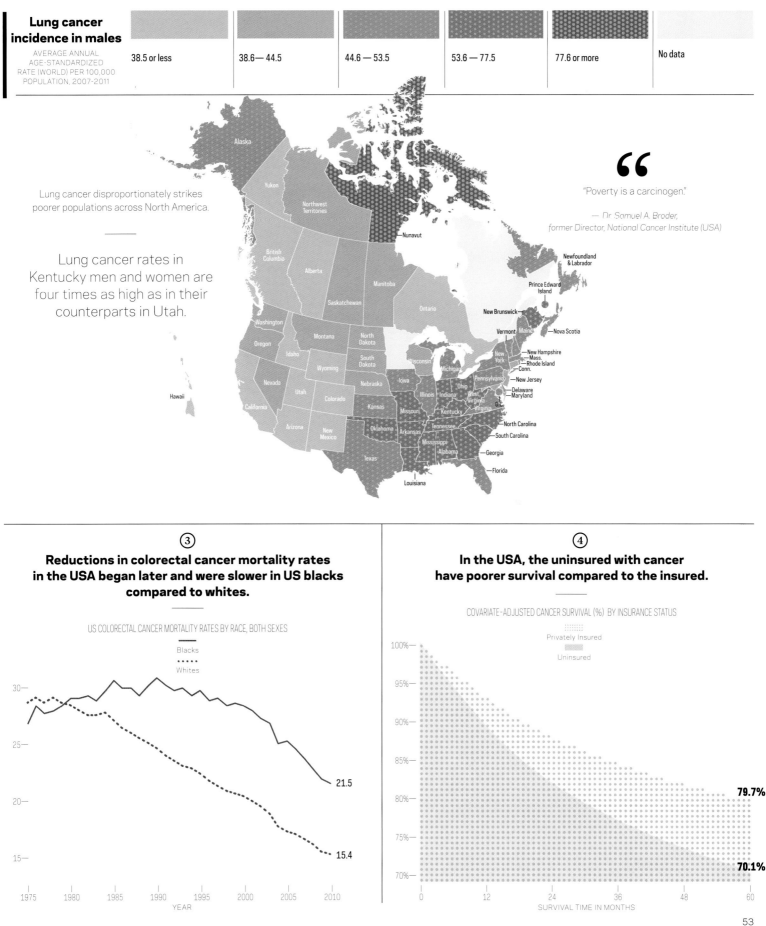

Lung cancer incidence in males

AVERAGE ANNUAL AGE-STANDARDIZED RATE (WORLD) PER 100,000 POPULATION, 2007-2011

| 38.5 or less | 38.6 — 44.5 | 44.6 — 53.5 | 53.6 — 77.5 | 77.6 or more | No data |

Lung cancer disproportionately strikes poorer populations across North America.

Lung cancer rates in Kentucky men and women are four times as high as in their counterparts in Utah.

"

"Poverty is a carcinogen."

— Dr. Samuel A. Broder,
former Director, National Cancer Institute (USA)

③

Reductions in colorectal cancer mortality rates in the USA began later and were slower in US blacks compared to whites.

US COLORECTAL CANCER MORTALITY RATES BY RACE, BOTH SEXES

Blacks
Whites

21.5

15.4

YEAR

④

In the USA, the uninsured with cancer have poorer survival compared to the insured.

COVARIATE-ADJUSTED CANCER SURVIVAL (%) BY INSURANCE STATUS

Privately Insured

Uninsured

79.7%

70.1%

SURVIVAL TIME IN MONTHS

REGIONAL DIVERSITY

Cancer in Southern, Eastern, and Southeastern Asia

Lung cancer is the leading cause of cancer deaths in this region; the other important cancers include oral cavity, stomach, breast, liver and colorectum.

This region, with 56% of the world's population (3.8 billion), contributes 44% of all cancer cases (6.4 million out of 14.1 million) and 51% of all cancer deaths (4.3 million out of 8.2 million) globally, with China representing the majority of the cancer burden. Incidence rates vary by almost fourfold, being highest in the Republic of Korea (307.8 per 100,000) and lowest in Bhutan (79.2 per 100,000), and mortality varies by threefold—from the highest in Mongolia (161 per 100,000) to the lowest in Maldives (53.7 per 100,000).

①️ In this region, the cancer burden is dominated by China. ②️ The top three cancers in women are breast, lung, and cervical cancers, while the top three causes of cancer death in women are lung, breast, and stomach cancer. In men the top three cancers are lung, stomach, and liver cancers, which are also the top three causes of cancer death.

③️ Due to changes in lifestyle and socio-cultural factors, a decreasing trend was observed for cervical cancer along with an increase in breast cancer in India, Thailand, China, and other countries. Oral cavity cancers are common in many southeastern and southern Asian countries due to the use of smokeless tobacco products. Although decreasing in many countries, stomach cancer rates remain high due to a high prevalence of *Helicobacter pylori* infection, and possibly due to dietary patterns.

Besides the universal modifiable cancer risk factors—tobacco use (smoking and chewable tobacco), unhealthy diet, physical inactivity and alcohol—infection with *H. pylori*, the liver fluke, indoor air pollution, and suboptimal immunization against hepatitis B are region-specific factors.

The regional burden of cancer is projected to increase by 41% (from 6.4 million in 2012 to 9 million by 2025) for incidence and 44% for mortality (from 4.3 million to 6.2 million), largely due to socio-economic growth and the increasing size and aging of the population. Therefore, it is critical that existing health systems are strengthened by appropriate policies and matching funding, not only to cope with the overall needs of treatment, but also to achieve maximal primary prevention and early detection of the most frequent treatable cancers.

①
China alone accounts for 50% of all cancer cases in this region.

TOP 5 COUNTRIES IN THIS REGION WITH THE HIGHEST ESTIMATED NUMBER OF CANCER CASES, 2012

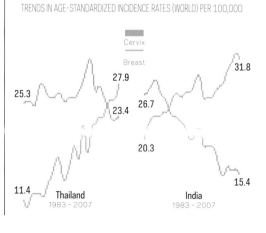

China **48.9%** 3,065,000 CASES

India **16.2%** 1,015,000 CASES

Japan **11.2%** 704,000 CASES

Indonesia **4.8%** 300,000 CASES

Rep. of Korea **3.5%** 220,000 CASES

②
Lung cancer has the highest incidence and mortality rates for both sexes combined.

ESTIMATED NUMBERS OF NEW CANCER CASES AND DEATHS, BOTH SEXES, 2012

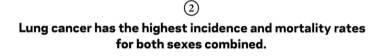

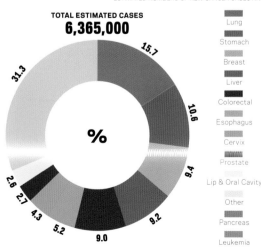

TOTAL ESTIMATED CASES 6,365,000

15.7 / 10.6 / 9.4 / 9.2 / 9.0 / 5.2 / 4.3 / 2.7 / 2.6 / 31.3

%

Lung
Stomach
Breast
Liver
Colorectal
Esophagus
Cervix
Prostate
Lip & Oral Cavity
Other
Pancreas
Leukemia

TOTAL ESTIMATED DEATHS 4,260,000

21.0 / 1.1 / 11.9 / 7.3 / 6.8 / 5.0 / 3.3 / 3.0 / 3.0 / 25.6

%

③
While cervical cancer has been decreasing in Thailand and India, breast cancer has been increasing and is now more common than cervical cancer.

TRENDS IN AGE-STANDARDIZED INCIDENCE RATES (WORLD) PER 100,000

Cervix
Breast

25.3 / 27.9 / 23.4 / 11.4
Thailand 1983 – 2007

31.8 / 26.7 / 20.3 / 15.4
India 1983 – 2007

Most commonly diagnosed cancers
2012

Colorectum	Lip & Oral Cavity	Stomach	Liver	Lung	Thyroid	Cervix	Breast
← MALE →			← BOTH SEXES →		← FEMALE →		
Fewest Countries | Most Countries			Fewest Countries | Most Countries		Fewest Countries | Most Countries		

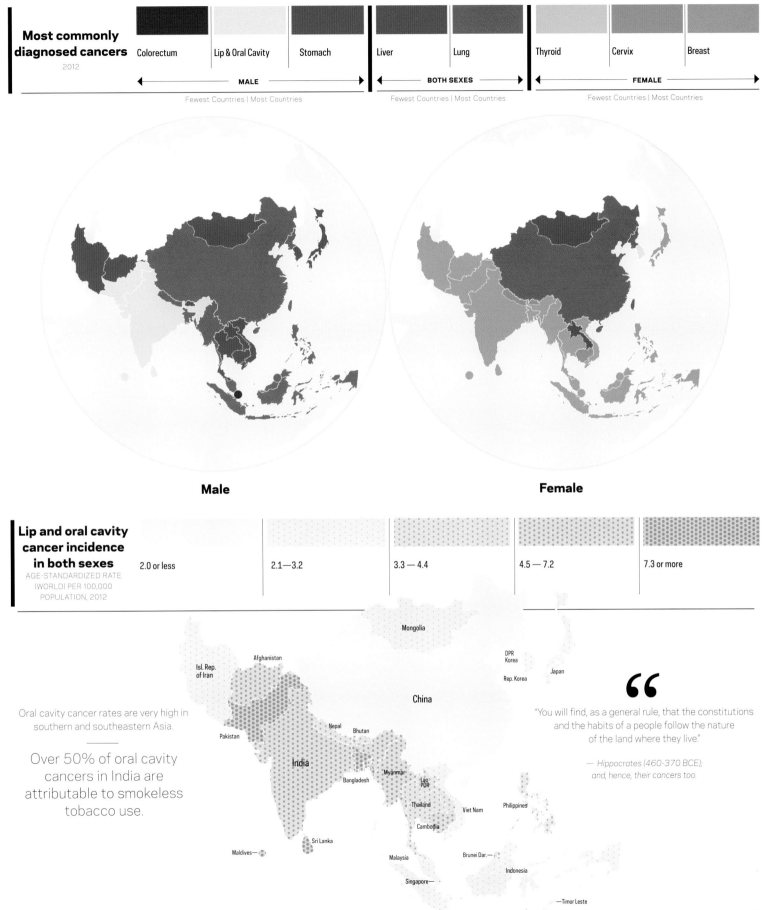

Male

Female

Lip and oral cavity cancer incidence in both sexes
AGE-STANDARDIZED RATE (WORLD) PER 100,000 POPULATION, 2012

2.0 or less	2.1 — 3.2	3.3 — 4.4	4.5 — 7.2	7.3 or more

Oral cavity cancer rates are very high in southern and southeastern Asia.

Over 50% of oral cavity cancers in India are attributable to smokeless tobacco use.

Mongolia

Afghanistan

Isl. Rep. of Iran

DPR Korea

Rep. Korea

Japan

China

Nepal

Pakistan

Bhutan

India

Myanmar

Bangladesh

Lao PDR

Thailand

Viet Nam

Philippines

Cambodia

Sri Lanka

Maldives—

Malaysia

Brunei Dar.—

Singapore—

Indonesia

—Timor Leste

"You will find, as a general rule, that the constitutions and the habits of a people follow the nature of the land where they live."

— *Hippocrates (460-370 BCE); and, hence, their cancers too.*

REGIONAL DIVERSITY

Cancer in Europe

Lung cancer is the most frequently diagnosed cancer in Europe, and also causes the most deaths in this region; other important cancers include breast, prostate, and colorectum.

Europe is characterized by striking geographical differences in cancer occurrence. There were an estimated 3.5 million new cancer cases and 1.9 million cancer deaths in Europe in 2012. ① Cancers of the female breast, colorectum, prostate and lung constitute over half of the overall incidence, while lung and colorectal cancer rank as the most common causes of cancer death.

In men, prostate cancer is the most frequent form of cancer incidence in most Northern, Western and Southern European countries, while lung cancer is the most frequently diagnosed cancer in Central and Eastern Europe. Lung cancer is the leading cause of cancer death among men in almost all European countries, while breast cancer dominates as the most frequent in women. ③ Lung cancer is also a leading cause of cancer death in certain European countries among women, overtaking breast cancer.

The variations in overall incidence rates across countries are three- to four-fold in men, and even greater in women. Current incidence and trends over 50 years reflect the different stages of the tobacco epidemic in different countries in men and women. ② In most European countries, lung cancer rates in men tend to have reached stability or are decreasing, while in women, they appear to be still increasing.

④ While breast cancer incidence rates continued to increase in most European countries, mortality rates decreased, as a result of earlier diagnosis and improved therapies. This effect is magnified among women of 50 years of age or older, the usual target of population-based screening programs in Europe.

"

"Cancer continues to present a huge challenge for patients, and their families, for health policy and for health services, across the European Union, and indeed beyond."

— Tonio Borg, European Commissioner for Health.

②

Lung cancer incidence rates vary greatly between European countries, in both men and women.

ESTIMATE AGE-STANDARDIZED INCIDENCE RATE (WORLD) OF LUNG CANCER IN EUROPE BY SEX, PER 100,000, 2012

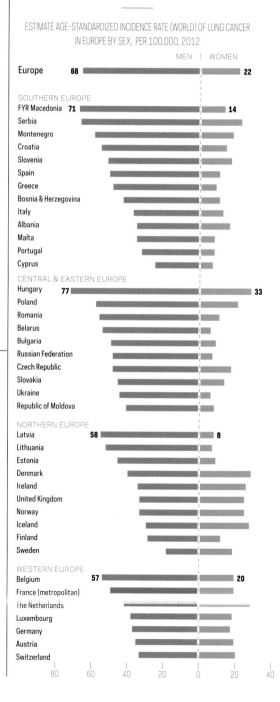

①

Cancers of the breast, colorectum, prostate and lung constitute over half of overall cancer incidence.

ESTIMATED NUMBERS OF NEW CANCER CASES AND DEATHS, BOTH SEXES, 2012

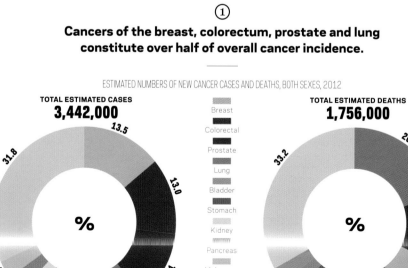

TOTAL ESTIMATED CASES
3,442,000
13.5
31.8
13.0
12.1
11.9
4.4
4.1
3.3
3.0
2.9

Breast
Colorectal
Prostate
Lung
Bladder
Stomach
Kidney
Pancreas
Melanoma
Other
Liver
Leukemia

TOTAL ESTIMATED DEATHS
1,756,000
20.1
33.2
12.2
7.5
6.1
6.0
5.3
3.5
3.1
3.0

Most commonly diagnosed cancers
2012

Colorectum	Lung	Prostate	Breast

◄———————————————————— MALE ————————————————————► | FEMALE

Fewest Countries | Most Countries

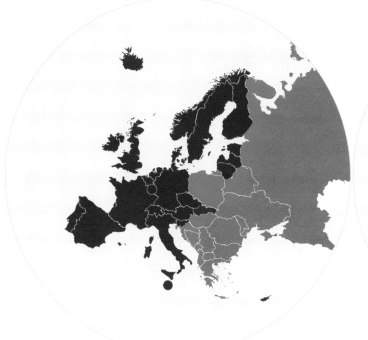
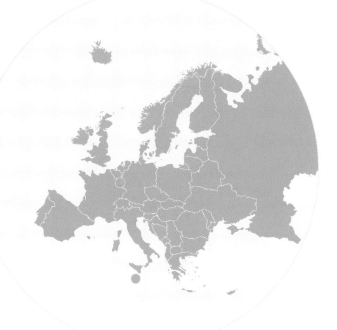

Male **Female**

---

③
Lung cancer now causes more deaths than breast cancer in some European countries.

———

TRENDS IN FEMALE LUNG AND BREAST CANCER AGE-STANDARDIZED MORTALITY RATES
(WORLD) PER 100,000 POPULATION, 1999-2011

Breast — United Kingdom
Lung ···· Poland

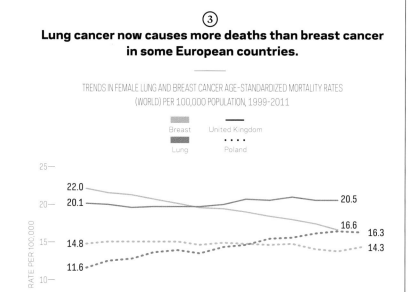

22.0
20.1
20.5
16.6
16.3
14.8
14.3
11.6

RATE PER 100,000
25—
20—
15—
10—
5—
0—

2000 2002 2004 2006 2008 2010

④
As a result of improved screening, earlier diagnosis and better therapies, breast cancer mortality decreased even as incidence increased in most European countries.

———

TRENDS IN AGE-STANDARDIZED INCIDENCE (WORLD) AND MORTALITY RATES
FOR BREAST CANCER IN WOMEN 50 YEARS OR OLDER

Incidence — The Netherlands
Mortality ···· Czech Republic

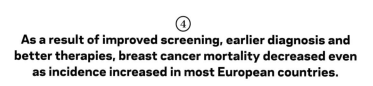
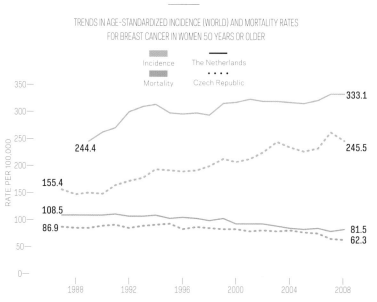

333.1
244.4
245.5
155.4
108.5
86.9
81.5
62.3

RATE PER 100,000
350—
300—
250—
200—
150—
100—
50—
0—

1988 1992 1996 2000 2004 2008

REGIONAL DIVERSITY

Cancer in Northern Africa and Central and Western Asia

In this region, lung cancer is the leading cause of cancer death among men, while breast cancer is the leading cause of cancer death among women.

Among the 492 million inhabitants of this region, 619,000 cancer cases and 383,000 cancer deaths occur each year, representing 4% and 5% of the worldwide cancer burden, respectively.

① In 2012, age-standardized rates per 100,000 population for all cancer sites (excluding non-melanoma skin cancers) for men and women were estimated to be 165 and 141 for incidence and 117 and 79 for mortality, respectively. Breast cancer is the most commonly diagnosed cancer in women, followed by colorectal and cervical cancer. In men, the three most commonly diagnosed cancers are lung, prostate, and bladder, and the three leading causes of cancer death are lung, liver, and stomach.

② The region is also characterized by marked variations in the incidence of various cancers, including high esophageal cancer incidence in Turkmenistan, Tajikistan, and Kazakhstan, high bladder cancer incidence in Lebanon, Turkey, Egypt, and several other countries of the region, and high liver cancer in Egypt. This region has some of the lowest cervical cancer rates in the world, although cervical cancer mortality rates have been rising among younger women in some West and Central Asian countries due to lack of effective screening and changing risk factors.

Within the next 20 years, the rapidly increasing population and aging are expected to double the new cancer cases and deaths from cancers; better detection, improved registration and increased prevalence of cancer risk factors will likely raise the numbers further.

③ Tobacco is among the most important of these risk factors. For example, Egypt has shown an increase in mortality from lung cancer.

The high liver cancer rate in Egypt is probably related to the high prevalence of chronic hepatitis C virus (HCV) infection, due to HCV-contaminated injection equipment used during mass treatment campaigns against *Schistosoma*; these same campaigns led to a sharp decline in squamous cell cancer of the urinary bladder. Poor nutrition, low fruit and vegetable intake, and drinking beverages at high temperatures have been proposed as possible explanations for the high esophageal cancer rates in Central Asia. Other important risk factors in the region include obesity, unhealthy diet, physical inactivity, air pollution, and increased exposure to industrial and agricultural carcinogens.

③

While bladder cancer mortality rates are decreasing in Egypt, other cancers are increasing, including colorectal, liver, lung, and breast cancers.

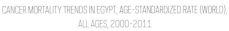

CANCER MORTALITY TRENDS IN EGYPT, AGE-STANDARDIZED RATE (WORLD), ALL AGES, 2000-2011

①

Lung and breast cancer are the most common diagnoses and causes of cancer death in this region, although there is substantial inter-regional variation in bladder, esophageal, and liver cancer incidence and mortality.

ESTIMATED NUMBERS OF NEW CANCER CASES AND DEATHS, BOTH SEXES, 2012

TOTAL ESTIMATED CASES
619,000

15.1 · 9.8 · 7.4 · 5.6 · 5.1 · 5.0 · 4.8 · 4.1 · 3.7 · 39.3

%

Legend: Breast · Lung · Colorectal · Bladder · Stomach · Prostate · Liver · NHL · Leukemia · Other

TOTAL ESTIMATED DEATHS
383,000

14.1 · 8.9 · 7.4 · 7.1 · 7.1 · 4.9 · 4.2 · 4.1 · 38.0

%

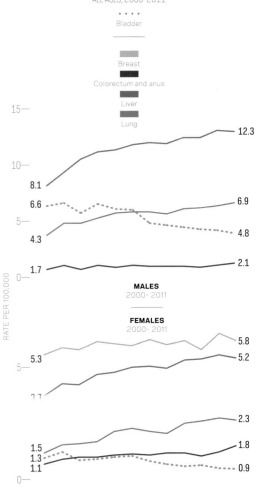

Most commonly diagnosed cancer among males
2012

Non-Hodgkin lymphoma	Liver	Leukemia	Prostate	Stomach	Colorectum	Lung

Fewest Countries ◄──► Most Countries

②

Bladder cancer incidence rates are strikingly high in some countries of this region, including Lebanon, Turkey, and Egypt.

ESTIMATED BLADDER CANCER INCIDENCE, AGE-STANDARDIZED RATE (WORLD), BOTH SEXES, 2012

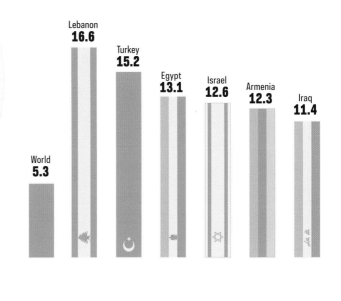

Lebanon **16.6**
Turkey **15.2**
Egypt **13.1**
Israel **12.6**
Armenia **12.3**
Iraq **11.4**
World **5.3**

The three most common cancers in males in this region— bladder, lung and liver—can largely be **prevented by tobacco control and anti-hepatitis measures.**

Esophageal cancer incidence in both sexes
ESTIMATED AGE-STANDARDIZED RATE (WORLD) PER 100,000 POPULATION, 2012

1.0 or less	1.1—1.7	1.8 — 3.6	3.7 — 10.1	10.2 or more

"

"Early detection of cancer and reliability of diagnoses are improving in the countries in the Gulf Corporation Council because of the availability of modern medical facilities. However, public awareness and education are not yet at a level that can affect diagnosis and control of cancers at the earliest stages."

—Dr. Robert Brown,
Department of Surgery and Cancer,
Imperial College London

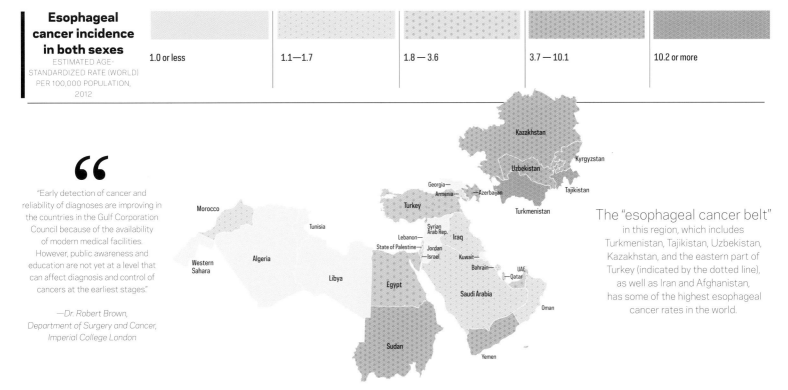

The "esophageal cancer belt" in this region, which includes Turkmenistan, Tajikistan, Uzbekistan, Kazakhstan, and the eastern part of Turkey (indicated by the dotted line), as well as Iran and Afghanistan, has some of the highest esophageal cancer rates in the world.

REGIONAL DIVERSITY

Cancer in Oceania

Oceania's three distinct sub-regions vary greatly in their cancer profiles (types of cancer and incidence and mortality rates).

① Oceania, a region that includes developed and transitioning economies, had an estimated 155,000 new cancers and 60,000 cancer deaths in 2012, with over 92% of the new cases and 87% of the deaths occurring in Australia and New Zealand (ANZ). The remaining cases and deaths occurred in the French Pacific (French Polynesia and New Caledonia) and the rest of Oceania (Papua New Guinea and many small island states), which are sparsely populated.

② The leading five cancers are prostate, colorectal, breast, melanoma, and lung in ANZ; prostate, breast, lung, colorectal, and thyroid in the French Pacific; and breast, cervix, oral cavity, liver, and lung in the rest of Oceania. These patterns are driven by variation in exposure to risk factors and in access to health services.

③ Lung cancer is the leading cause of cancer death within Oceania. Since the 1980s, lung cancer mortality among men has declined in Australia because of substantial declines in the prevalence of smoking. In contrast, rates continue to increase among women because of the lag in smoking reduction.

Incidence rates of breast cancer in ANZ are up to four times higher than in other countries in Oceania because of reproductive factors and mammography utilization (see chapter 12 – *Breast Cancer*). ⑤ ⑥ In contrast, cervix and liver cancers are more common in areas of Oceania other than ANZ. These cancers are linked to a high prevalence of human papillomavirus and hepatitis B infections. Organized screening for cervix cancer in Australia has achieved a decline in incidence.

⑦ Melanoma varies 35-fold, with ANZ rates around 35 per 100,000. ANZ has the highest incidence globally due to people of European descent being exposed to high levels of solar radiation. Within Australia, incidence varies with latitude.

---

①

Cancer patterns in Oceania are driven by the large populations of high-income countries Australia and New Zealand.

ESTIMATED NUMBERS OF NEW CANCER CASES AND DEATHS, BOTH SEXES, 2012

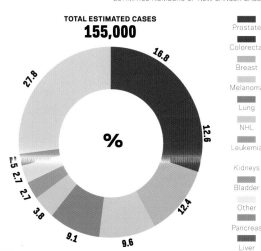
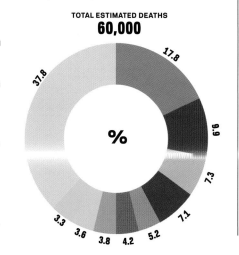

---

②

The three sub-regions of Oceania vary markedly in risk factors and treatment availability, resulting in diverse cancer profiles.

ESTIMATED TOTAL CANCER CASES AND CONTRIBUTION OF TOP 5 CANCER SITES BY SUBREGION, BOTH SEXES, 2012

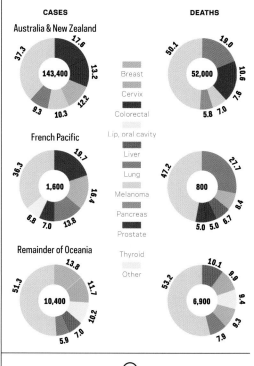

---

③

The different lung cancer mortality trends observed by sex reflect the fact that smoking prevalence has been declining for Australian men since 1945 and for women since 1980.

TRENDS IN AGE-STANDARDIZED LUNG CANCER MORTALITY RATES PER 100,000 POPULATION AND SMOKING PREVALENCE (%), 1945-2010

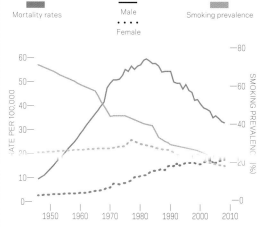

Cervical cancer incidence rate

ESTIMATED AGE-STANDARDIZED RATE (WORLD) PER 100,000, 2012

9.0 or less	9.1—19.2	19.3 or more

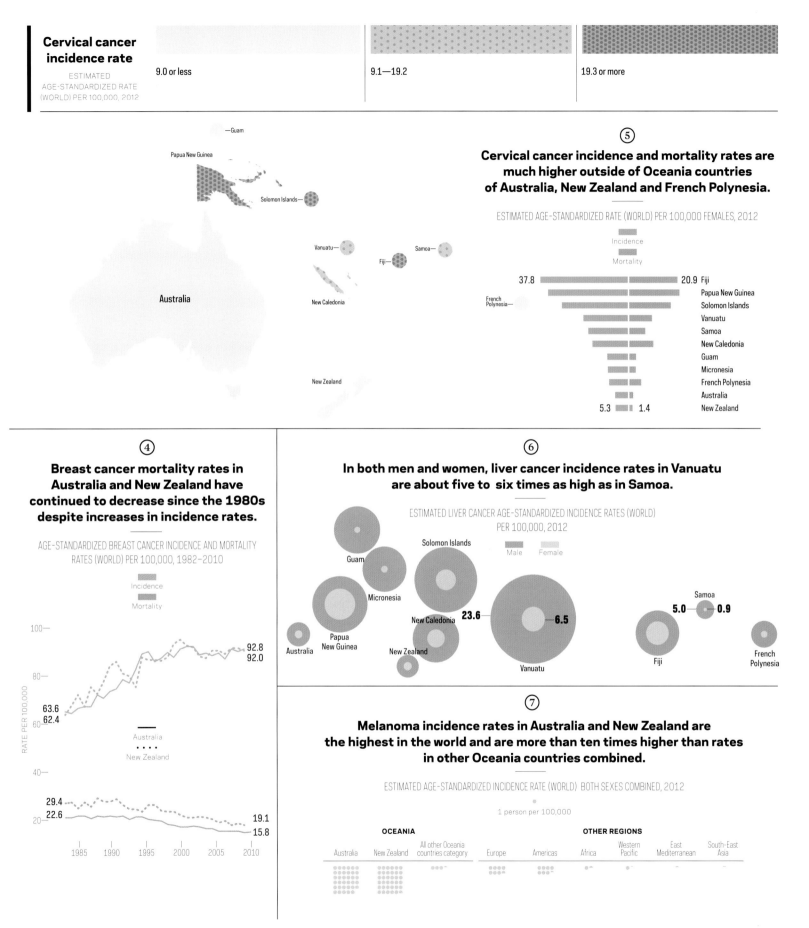

—Guam

Papua New Guinea

Solomon Islands—

Vanuatu—

Fiji—

Samoa—

New Caledonia

Australia

New Zealand

⑤ Cervical cancer incidence and mortality rates are much higher outside of Oceania countries of Australia, New Zealand and French Polynesia.

ESTIMATED AGE-STANDARDIZED RATE (WORLD) PER 100,000 FEMALES, 2012

Incidence

Mortality

French Polynesia—

37.8		20.9	Fiji
			Papua New Guinea
			Solomon Islands
			Vanuatu
			Samoa
			New Caledonia
			Guam
			Micronesia
			French Polynesia
			Australia
5.3		1.4	New Zealand

④ Breast cancer mortality rates in Australia and New Zealand have continued to decrease since the 1980s despite increases in incidence rates.

AGE-STANDARDIZED BREAST CANCER INCIDENCE AND MORTALITY RATES (WORLD) PER 100,000, 1982–2010

Incidence

Mortality

100—

92.8
92.0

80—

63.6
62.4

RATE PER 100,000

Australia

New Zealand

40—

29.4

20— 22.6

19.1
15.8

1985   1990   1995   2000   2005   2010

⑥ In both men and women, liver cancer incidence rates in Vanuatu are about five to six times as high as in Samoa.

ESTIMATED LIVER CANCER AGE-STANDARDIZED INCIDENCE RATES (WORLD) PER 100,000, 2012

Male   Female

Guam

Solomon Islands

Micronesia

New Caledonia

Papua New Guinea

Australia

New Zealand

23.6   6.5

Vanuatu

5.0   0.9   Samoa

Fiji

French Polynesia

⑦ Melanoma incidence rates in Australia and New Zealand are the highest in the world and are more than ten times higher than rates in other Oceania countries combined.

ESTIMATED AGE-STANDARDIZED INCIDENCE RATE (WORLD) BOTH SEXES COMBINED, 2012

1 person per 100,000

OCEANIA			OTHER REGIONS					
Australia	New Zealand	All other Oceania countries category	Europe	Americas	Africa	Western Pacific	East Mediterranean	South-East Asia

CANCER SURVIVORSHIP

It is estimated that in 2012, there were 32.6 million people living who had been diagnosed with cancer within the previous five years.

① There are more cancer survivors living in more developed regions (17 million) than less-developed regions (15.6 million), although more cases are diagnosed in low- and middle-income countries. This reflects improved survival, related to higher rates of early detection and better access to effective treatment in high-income countries.

② Among men diagnosed in the past five years, over a quarter of all cancer survivors have had a diagnosis of prostate cancer, after which colorectal cancer (13%) and lung cancer (8%) were the most common sites diagnosed.

Among women, breast cancer survivors make the largest contribution, constituting over a third of all those living with a cancer diagnosis in the past five years. This is followed by colorectal and cervical cancers, each with 9% of the total.

Estimated distribution of 5-year population prevalence for all cancers combined, excluding non-melanoma skin cancer

NUMBER OF SURVIVORS DIAGNOSED WITHIN THE PAST FIVE YEARS PER 100,000 ADULTS (15+ YEARS), BOTH SEXES, 2012

"

"The story of cancer…isn't the story of doctors who struggle and survive, moving from institution to another. It is the story of patients who struggle and survive, moving from one embankment of illness to another. Resilience, inventiveness, and survivorship—qualities often ascribed to great physicians—are reflected qualities, emanating first from those who struggle with illness."

— Siddhartha Mukherjee, The Emperor of All Maladies

①

In countries at high or very high levels of the Human Development Index, the proportion of the population who are cancer survivors is much higher than in countries at low or medium levels, although the profile of such survivors varies by Index level.

ESTIMATED 5-YEAR CANCER PREVALENCE PROPORTIONS (NUMBER OF SURVIVORS DIAGNOSED WITHIN THE PAST FIVE YEARS PER 500,000 POPULATION) IN ADULT MEN AND WOMEN (>15 YEARS), BY HUMAN DEVELOPMENT INDEX FOR SELECT CANCER SITES, 2012

● 1 survivor per 20,000 population

MEN	Prostate	Colorectal	Lung	Stomach	Bladder	Liver	Lip, oral cavity	Kaposi sarcoma	Other pharynx
Very High HDI									
High HDI									
Medium HDI									
Low HDI									

WOMEN	Breast	Colorectal	Lung	Corpus uteri	Cervix	Thyroid	Ovary
Very High HDI							
High HDI							
Medium HDI							
Low HDI							

Almost 1 in 5 cancer survivors in the world diagnosed within the past five years is a woman who has had breast cancer.

Canada

United States of America

Mexico

Bahamas
Cuba
Haiti
Dominican Rep.
Belize
Jamaica
Honduras
Puerto Rico
Guatemala
El Salvador
Nicaragua
Guadeloupe
Martinique
Barbados
Trinidad & Tobago
Costa Rica
Panama
Venezuela
Guyana
French Guiana
Colombia
Suriname
Ecuador
Peru
Brazil
Bolivia
Paraguay
Argentina
Uruguay
Chile

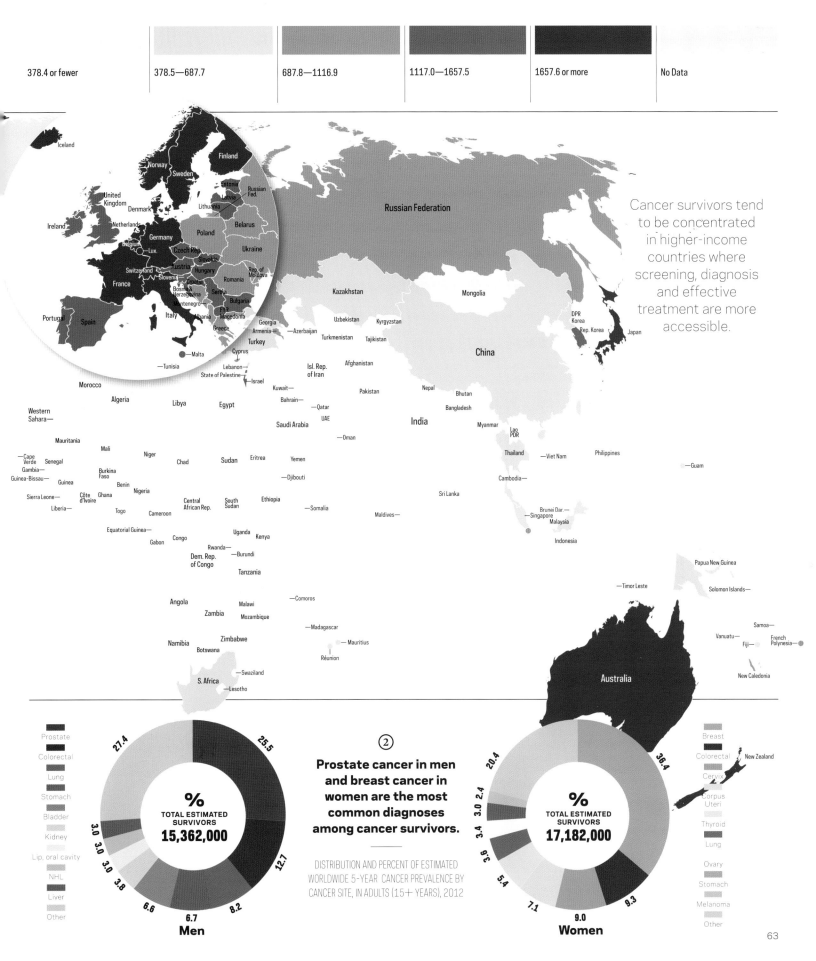

378.4 or fewer | 378.5—687.7 | 687.8—1116.9 | 1117.0—1657.5 | 1657.6 or more | No Data

Cancer survivors tend to be concentrated in higher-income countries where screening, diagnosis and effective treatment are more accessible.

② Prostate cancer in men and breast cancer in women are the most common diagnoses among cancer survivors.

DISTRIBUTION AND PERCENT OF ESTIMATED WORLDWIDE 5-YEAR CANCER PREVALENCE BY CANCER SITE, IN ADULTS (15+ YEARS), 2012

Men

%
TOTAL ESTIMATED SURVIVORS
15,362,000

Prostate — 25.5
Colorectal — 12.7
Lung — 8.2
Stomach — 6.7
Bladder — 6.6
Kidney — 3.8
Lip, oral cavity — 3.0
NHL — 3.0
Liver — 3.0
Other — 27.4

Women

%
TOTAL ESTIMATED SURVIVORS
17,182,000

Breast — 36.4
Colorectal — 9.3
Cervix — 9.0
Corpus Uteri — 7.1
Thyroid — 5.4
Lung — 3.6
Ovary — 3.4
Stomach — 3.0
Melanoma — 2.4
Other — 20.4

63

TAKING ACTION

"

There are several advantages to primary prevention, including:
(...) the effectiveness may have benefits beyond those directly exposed;
avoidance of exposure to carcinogenic agents is likely
to prevent other non-communicable diseases;
and the cause may be removed or reduced long-term,
(...) i.e. the preventive effort does not need to be renewed
with every generation. This is especially important when
resources are in short supply.

— *Vineis and Wild*, Lancet, 2014

Prevention

—

Primary prevention is a particularly effective way to fight cancer, with between one third and one half of cancers being preventable based on current knowledge of risk factors.

PROPORTION OF CANCERS THAT CAN BE PREVENTED WITH CURRENT KNOWLEDGE

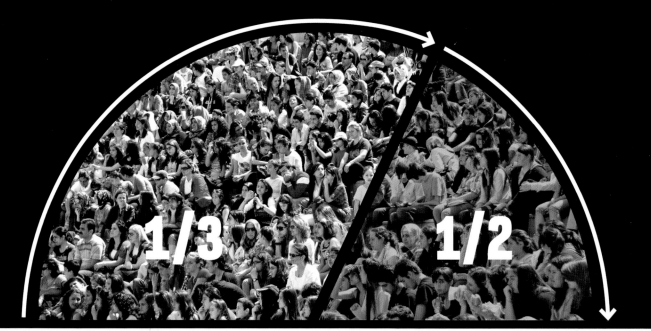

1/3   1/2

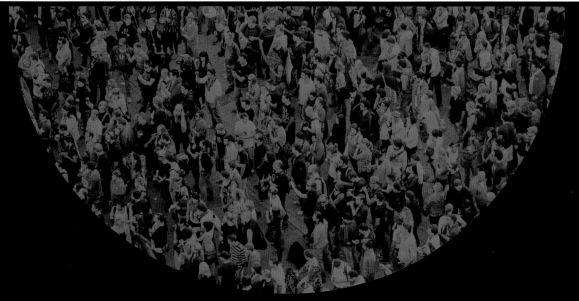

THE CANCER CONTINUUM

An overview of interventions and potential for impact:

Opportunities for cancer control exist at all stages of the cancer continuum, from preventing cancer to developing and providing adequate palliative care.

(1) Interventions for cancer prevention and control at the individual and population levels exist across the cancer continuum from prevention of risk factors to early detection, treatment and palliative care. (2) Tobacco use, the cause of the most preventable cancers worldwide, can be substantially reduced through increased excise tax on cigarettes, smoke-free air laws, restrictions on promotion, and counter-advertising. Indoor and outdoor air pollution, which account for a substantial proportion of lung cancer deaths, can be reduced through use of clean stoves, cleaner fuels, proper ventilation, and air quality guidelines and policies. (3) Vaccines against Hepatitis B virus and human papillomaviruses could reduce the future burden of liver and cervical cancers,

"An ounce of prevention is worth a pound of cure."

— Benjamin Franklin

respectively, particularly in economically developing countries. Furthermore, transmission of these and some other cancer causing agents (e.g., *Schistosoma haematobium*, hepatitis C virus) can be prevented by improving hygiene and educating people to modify their high risk behaviors. Protection from harmful sun exposure reduces the risk of skin cancer. Cancer-causing occupational exposures can be prevented through improved workplace safety.

Regular screening for cervical, colorectal, and breast cancers detects the disease at an early stage, when the chance for survival and cure is high. A heightened awareness of warning signs for cancer of the oral cavity, skin, and some other cancers may also lead to detection of cancers at an early stage.

(4) Effective treatment (surgery, chemotherapy, and radiation) has been developed for several cancers, including cancers of the breast, colon and rectum, and testis and for many childhood cancers. For certain cancers such as testis, treatment could lead to cure even for advanced stage disease. Pain associated with cancer can be controlled by administration of analgesic drugs. Full application of these interventions globally could prevent a substantial proportion of cancer deaths worldwide.

(1)
Interventions for cancer prevention and control at the individual and population levels exist across the cancer continuum.

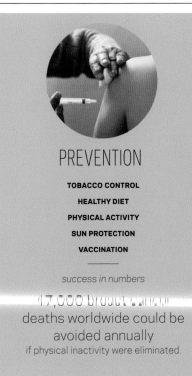

PREVENTION

TOBACCO CONTROL

HEALTHY DIET

PHYSICAL ACTIVITY

SUN PROTECTION

VACCINATION

success in numbers

~~17,000 breast cancer~~
deaths worldwide could be avoided annually
if physical inactivity were eliminated.

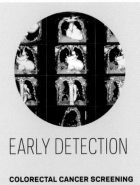

EARLY DETECTION

COLORECTAL CANCER SCREENING

BREAST CANCER SCREENING

CERVICAL CANCER SCREENING

success in numbers

Biennial colorectal cancer screening using the fecal occult blood test, a low-cost method, can result in
a 15–20% decrease in colorectal cancer mortality.

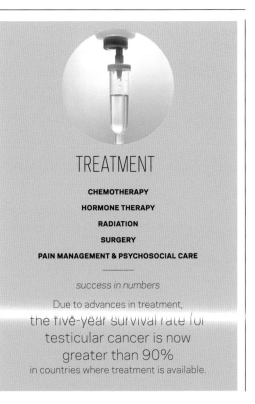

TREATMENT

CHEMOTHERAPY

HORMONE THERAPY

RADIATION

SURGERY

PAIN MANAGEMENT & PSYCHOSOCIAL CARE

success in numbers

Due to advances in treatment,
the five-year survival rate for testicular cancer is now greater than 90%
in countries where treatment is available.

② Smoking cessation is beneficial at all ages, but especially before middle age.

PROBABILITY OF DEATH FROM LUNG CANCER BY ATTAINED AGE

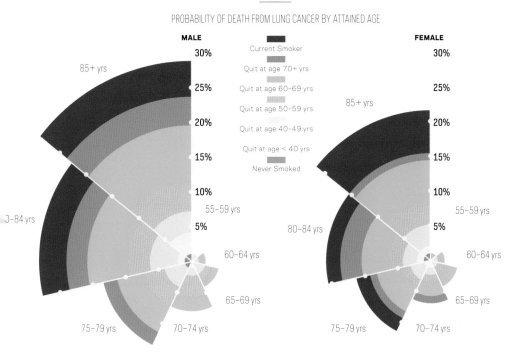

MALE

FEMALE

Current Smoker
Quit at age 70+ yrs
Quit at age 60-69 yrs
Quit at age 50-59 yrs
Quit at age 40-49 yrs
Quit at age < 40 yrs
Never Smoked

A 70% price increase on tobacco along with a 10% reduction in consumption through other tobacco control measures would avoid 25 million cancer deaths by 2050.

③ Cervical cancer deaths are preventable.

NUMBER OF FUTURE DEATHS THAT COULD BE PREVENTED IN ONE YEAR IF 70% OF 9-YEAR-OLD GIRLS WERE VACCINATED

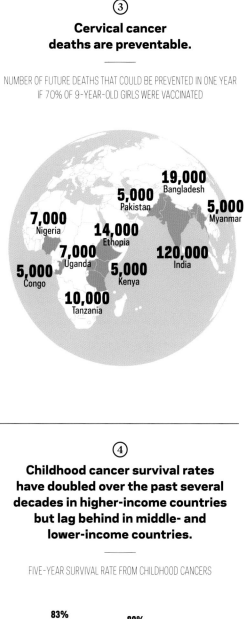

④ Childhood cancer survival rates have doubled over the past several decades in higher-income countries but lag behind in middle- and lower-income countries.

FIVE-YEAR SURVIVAL RATE FROM CHILDHOOD CANCERS

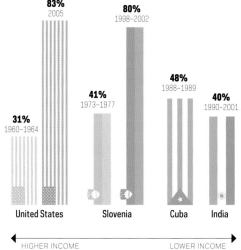

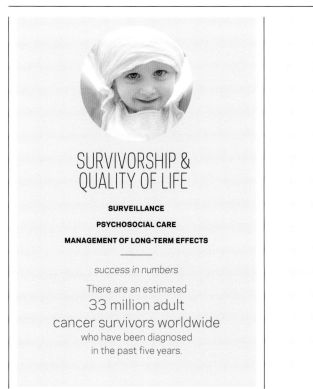

SURVIVORSHIP & QUALITY OF LIFE

SURVEILLANCE

PSYCHOSOCIAL CARE

MANAGEMENT OF LONG-TERM EFFECTS

success in numbers

There are an estimated 33 million adult cancer survivors worldwide who have been diagnosed in the past five years.

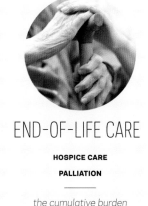

END-OF-LIFE CARE

HOSPICE CARE

PALLIATION

the cumulative burden

Cancer accounts for 34% of the adult palliative care needs in the world.

HEALTH PROMOTION

A population and systems approach:

The key to reducing cancer lies in prevention, not in cure.

Because of the rising cost of treating illness coupled with the difficult economic environment, interest in health promotion is increasing worldwide. The World Health Organization (WHO) defines health promotion as the process of enabling people to increase control over their health and its determinants (e.g. smoking, physical activity, diet), and thereby improve their health. ① This is usually addressed by activities aimed at promoting healthy behaviors and creating healthy policies and environments in order to affect large segments of the population. ② The impact of these activities is enhanced if healthy public policy is adopted across all sectors of society, especially by governments, including in settings such as urban planning not typically seen as part of the health system.

The WHO Health Promoting Schools initiative aims to prevent tobacco use, sedentary lifestyles, and unhealthy nutrition worldwide. In many countries, education on these risk factors is part of the school curriculum. Instilling healthy behaviors and practices during youth may be easier and more effective than changing entrenched unhealthy behaviors during adulthood.

Many employers, especially in high-income countries, have health promotion programs for their workers, since such programs have been shown to increase productivity and reduce costs. Governments as well as public and private health organizations also play pivotal roles in motivating people to adopt healthy lifestyles and increasing awareness about cancer. For example, several countries have banned smoking in public places and require health warnings on cigarettes or nutrition labels on foods. The Union for International Cancer Control holds World Cancer Day each February to improve awareness about cancer and healthy behaviors.

② **Health promotion includes not only health education for individual-level behaviors, but also actions in all sectors of society, including communities and governments.**

HEALTH PROMOTION STRATEGIES

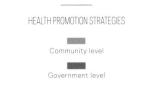

Community level

Government level

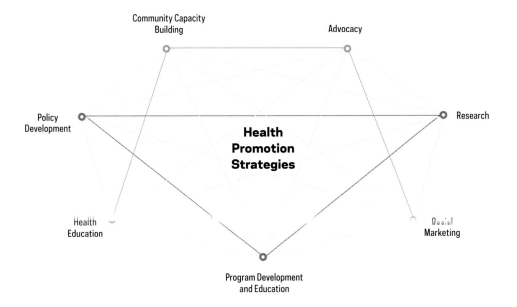

Community Capacity Building

Advocacy

Policy Development

Research

Health Promotion Strategies

Health Education

Social Marketing

Program Development and Education

① **Social marketing campaigns promoting physical activity increase class attendance.**

AVERAGE MONTHLY ATTENDANCE AT PHYSICAL ACTIVITY SESSIONS SUPPORTED BY FIT 'N FAB SOCIAL MARKETING PROGRAM COMPARED TO PRE-EXISTING SESSIONS WITHOUT SOCIAL MARKETING, SOUTHMEAD, BRISTOL, UK

Pre-existing gym classes

Social marketing intervention classes

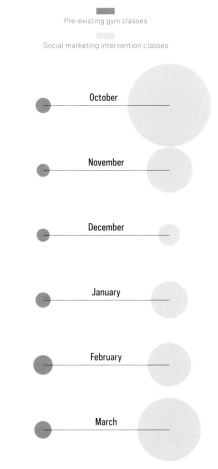

October

November

December

January

February

March

A six-month social marketing campaign to promote physical activity in a low-income area of the United Kingdom resulted in higher class attendance than at the pre-existing classes not related to the social marketing program.

The WHO's Global School Health Initiative has established Health Promoting School Programmes in all six WHO regions, including the 11 most populous countries in the world (Bangladesh, Brazil, China, India, Indonesia, Japan, Mexico, Nigeria, Pakistan, Russian Federation, USA).

Warning labels on cigarette packaging

WHO FCTC, 2013

Large with all appropriate characteristics	Medium or large but missing appropriate characteristics	None or small	No Data

Many countries have adopted at least some warning labels for cigarette packaging, although in many cases they lack all of the proven-effective characteristics specified by the WHO FCTC:

1.
Describe the harmful effects of tobacco use

2.
Be approved by the appropriate national authority

3.
Appear on at least 30%, and ideally 50% or more, of the package's principal display areas

4.
Be large, clear, visible, and legible in the country's principal language(s)

5.
Have multiple, rotating messages

6.
Use pictures or pictograms

Nutrition label policies

UNITED NATIONS FOOD AND AGRICULTURE ORGANIZATION, 2010

Mandatory	Voluntary	No Data

Food nutrition labels are becoming common around the world, particularly in

high-income countries.

"The function of protecting and developing health must rank even above that of restoring it when it is impaired."

— *Hippocrates*

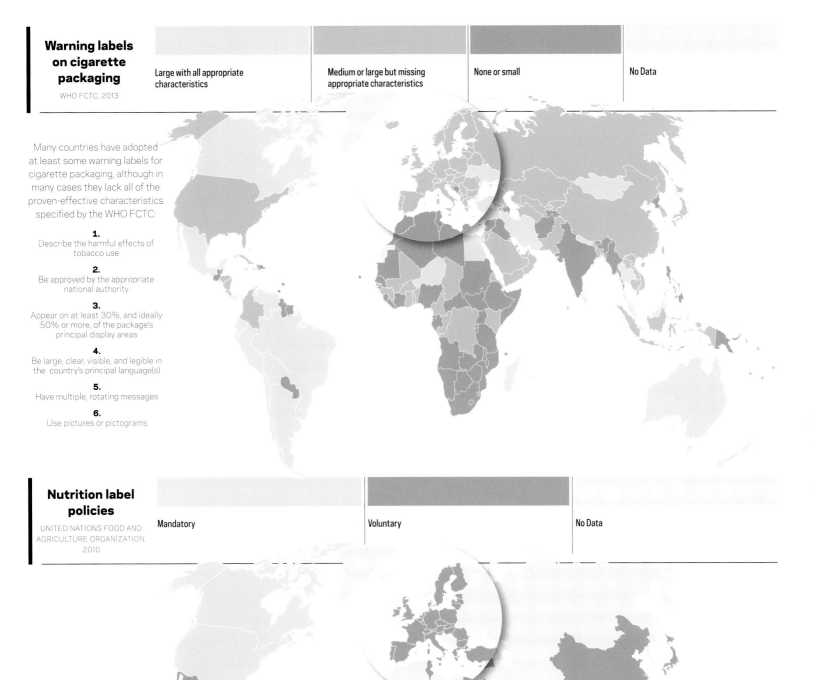

TOBACCO CONTROL

Tobacco control measures can reduce tobacco use, which is one of the most significant causes of cancer today.

Tobacco use is the cause of the most preventable cancer deaths, and in many countries, the leading cause of cancer death. Furthermore, it is a risk factor that is the most globalized, and as such it has elicited a global response through the World Health Organization (WHO).

The cornerstone of tobacco control policies is the WHO Framework Convention on Tobacco Control (FCTC), its Guidelines, and the Illicit Trade Protocol. The WHO FCTC is the only treaty negotiated under the auspices of the WHO, and includes 179 Parties.

The treaty entered into force in February 2005 and provides an internationally coordinated response to combating the tobacco epidemic with specific steps for governments addressing tobacco use. These include demand reduction measures such as adopting tax and price measures to reduce tobacco consumption; banning tobacco advertising, promotion, and sponsorship; creating smoke-free work and public spaces; placing health warnings on tobacco packages; and supply reduction measures such as combating the illicit trade in tobacco products.

The most widely implemented tobacco control policies are focused on reducing the demand for tobacco products, thereby decreasing consumption and prevalence by reducing initiation (prevention) or increasing cessation (intervention). (1)(2) Tax and price policies are often cited as the most effective demand-sided policy, because taxes are able to be increased on a regular and consistent basis. Evidence in Brazil, Thailand, and South Africa suggests that increases in taxes and price were the largest contributors to the decline in tobacco use.

Tobacco control policies must ensure that tax increases result in tobacco product price increases of such magnitude that the affordability of tobacco products declines. Over the last 20 years, tobacco products have become less affordable in high-income countries because of tax and price increases, and because incomes have not been growing rapidly. (3) However, the opposite has been seen in low- and middle-income countries where cigarettes have become more affordable because taxes and prices have been rising more slowly than increases in incomes.

In 2008, WHO introduced the MPOWER measures to assist in country-level implementation of the WHO FCTC provisions.

MPOWER MEASURES

M
MONITOR tobacco use and prevention policies

P
PROTECT people from tobacco smoke

O
OFFER help to quit tobacco use

W
WARN about the dangers of tobacco

E
ENFORCE bans on tobacco advertising, promotion, and sponsorship

R
RAISE taxes on tobacco

"

"Tobacco is the only industry that produces products to make huge profits and at the same time damage the health and kill their consumers."

— *Dr. Margaret Chan*
Director-General of the World Health Organization

Tobacco control measures are estimated to have contributed to substantial decreases in smoking and smoking-related deaths.

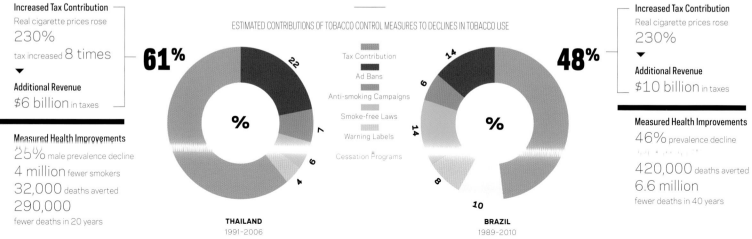

ESTIMATED CONTRIBUTIONS OF TOBACCO CONTROL MEASURES TO DECLINES IN TOBACCO USE

Increased Tax Contribution
Real cigarette prices rose
230%
tax increased 8 times
▼
Additional Revenue
$6 billion in taxes

Measured Health Improvements
25% male prevalence decline
4 million fewer smokers
32,000 deaths averted
290,000
fewer deaths in 20 years

61%

Tax Contribution
Ad Bans
Anti-smoking Campaigns
Smoke-free Laws
Warning Labels
Cessation Programs

22
7
6
4

48%

14
9
14
8
10

Increased Tax Contribution
Real cigarette prices rose
230%
▼
Additional Revenue
$10 billion in taxes

Measured Health Improvements
46% prevalence decline
420,000 deaths averted
6.6 million
fewer deaths in 40 years

THAILAND
1991–2006

BRAZIL
1989–2010

Parties to the WHO FCTC

Parties

Non-Parties

No Data

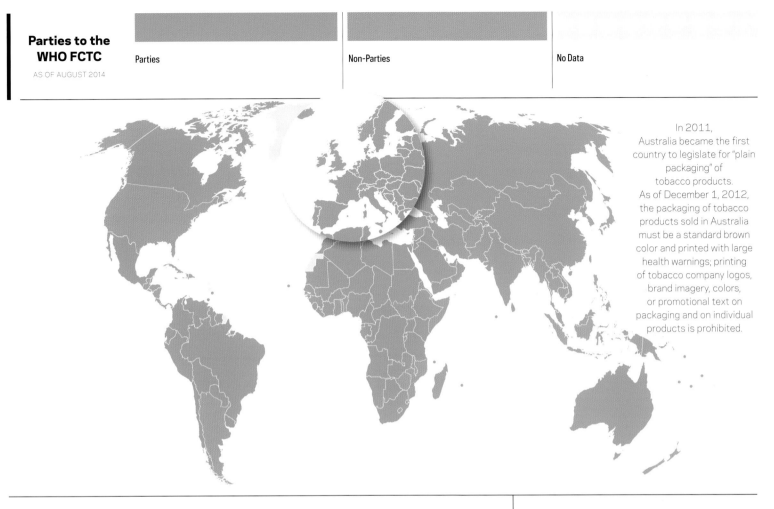

In 2011, Australia became the first country to legislate for "plain packaging" of tobacco products. As of December 1, 2012, the packaging of tobacco products sold in Australia must be a standard brown color and printed with large health warnings; printing of tobacco company logos, brand imagery, colors, or promotional text on packaging and on individual products is prohibited.

---

②

In South Africa, as cigarettes became less affordable, cigarette consumption began to decrease.

CIGARETTE PRICES, AFFORDABILITY, AND CONSUMPTION IN SOUTH AFRICA, 1961-2012

RELATIVE INCOME PRICE
% of per-capita GDP required to purchase 100 packs of cigarettes

CONSUMPTION
packs per person per annum

REAL RETAIL PRICE
Rands per 20 cigarettes

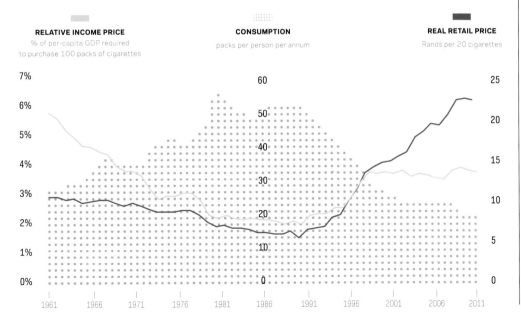

③

In low- and middle-income countries, cigarettes have become more affordable because taxes and prices have been rising more slowly than increases in incomes.

CUMULATIVE CHANGE IN CIGARETTE AFFORDABILITY
(PERCENT OF INCOME REQUIRED TO PURCHASE CIGARETTES), 1990-2006

IN LOW & MIDDLE-INCOME COUNTRIES, cigarettes became relatively MORE affordable.

25%

-27%

IN HIGH-INCOME COUNTRIES, cigarettes became relatively LESS affordable.

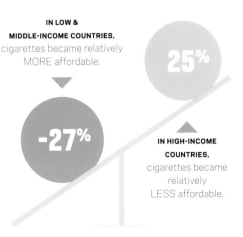

VACCINES

Highly effective
and safe vaccines
are available to
prevent HBV and
HPV infections and
associated cancers.

Hepatitis B virus (HBV) infection causes over 750,000 deaths annually, including 340,000 cases of hepatocellular carcinoma (HCC) globally. HCC results from chronic HBV infection, and the risk of chronic infection is greatest if transmission occurs during birth and early childhood. Highly effective vaccines for hepatitis B have been available since 1982 as a 3-dose series. To prevent mother-to-child transmission, the first dose should be given within 24 hours of birth, and at least two additional doses should be included as part of routine childhood vaccination. Through mid-2013, 181 countries had introduced hepatitis B vaccination. Globally, 3-dose vaccination coverage among children reached 75%, but less than half of the countries report offering a birth dose. Hepatitis B vaccination is estimated to avert over 700,000 future HBV deaths for every vaccinated birth cohort globally.

① Human papillomavirus (HPV) is the cause of 610,000 cancers annually, 87% of which are cervical cancers, 9.5% other anogenital and 3.5% oropharyngeal. Two HPV vaccines have been available since 2006; both are highly effective and safe, and protect against HPV types 16 and 18—types that cause over 70% of all cervical cancers and the majority of other cancers that are caused by HPV. The vaccines are given as a 3-dose or a 2-dose series. The target group for HPV vaccination is young adolescent girls in most countries. A few countries also recommend vaccination for boys. The first countries to introduce HPV vaccine were high-income countries, due to the cost of vaccines. Middle- and low-income countries started to introduce HPV vaccine 3-6 years later. By mid-2013, 45 countries had introduced HPV vaccination.

①

HPV accounts for an important proportion of cases for some cancer sites; for cervical cancer, virtually all cases are attributable to HPV infection.

PERCENTAGE OF CANCER CASES ATTRIBUTABLE TO HPV INFECTION WORLDWIDE AND TOTAL NUMBER OF NEW CASES, 2008

Number of cases not attributable to HPV

Number of cases attributable to HPV

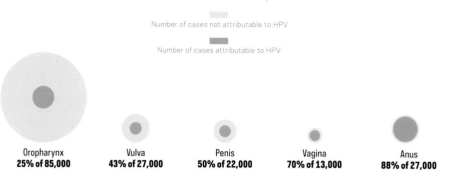

Oropharynx	Vulva	Penis	Vagina	Anus
25% of 85,000	**43% of 27,000**	**50% of 22,000**	**70% of 13,000**	**88% of 27,000**

Cervix
Nearly 100% of 530,000 Cases

Cervical cancer accounts for a smaller proportion of all HPV attributable cancers in countries with cervical cancer screening programs.

Countries that have introduced the HPV vaccine

2013

Have introduced HPV vaccine by 2013

No HPV vaccine introduced as of 2013

No Data

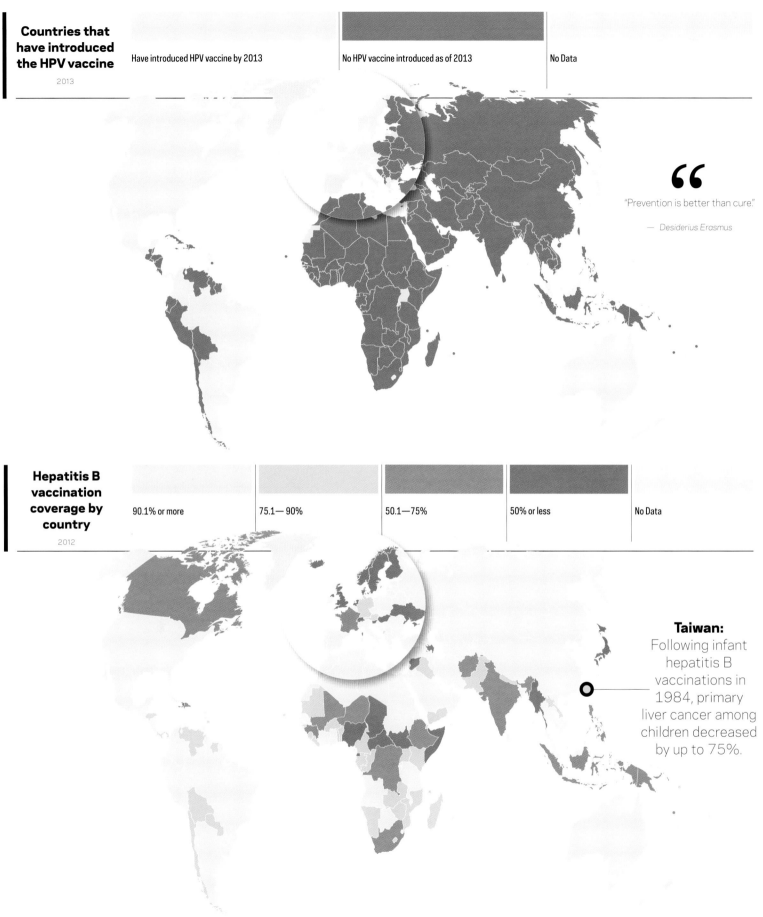

"
"Prevention is better than cure."

— *Desiderius Erasmus*

Hepatitis B vaccination coverage by country

2012

90.1% or more

75.1— 90%

50.1—75%

50% or less

No Data

Taiwan: Following infant hepatitis B vaccinations in 1984, primary liver cancer among children decreased by up to 75%.

EARLY DETECTION

Early detection is an essential component of cancer control.

Cancer early detection involves detecting cancers at early stages when they can be effectively treated and cured. Improved awareness among the general public and health care providers of early cancer, as well as good access to effective health services, can lead to earlier clinical diagnosis and prompt treatment. Screening programs for asymptomatic, apparently healthy populations are resource-intensive interventions, and should be undertaken only when their effectiveness has been demonstrated, when health services are adequately developed to investigate, treat and follow up screen-positive individuals, and when there is a sufficiently high incidence of the disease to justify the effort and costs of screening.

① Screening programs vary between countries in how they are conducted; they are more organized in countries such as Australia, Finland and the United Kingdom among others with systematic call and recall of target populations at regular intervals, compared with unorganized programs in countries such as the United States, France, and Germany.

② Pap smear screening programs have substantially reduced cervical cancer incidence and mortality in several high-income countries. Alternative cervical screening tests include human papillomavirus (HPV) testing and visual inspection with acetic acid (VIA). HPV testing is shown to be more sensitive than the pap smear in detecting cervical neoplasia, and VIA is a feasible and effective intervention in low-income countries. Mammography screening and treatment improvements have reduced breast cancer deaths in many high-income countries. It is unclear whether clinical breast examination screening can reduce breast cancer mortality. Screening with fecal occult blood tests has reduced colorectal cancer mortality in clinical trials, and organized colorectal cancer screening programs are still evolving in high-income countries. Oral cancer screening, using visual inspection, has been shown to reduce oral cancer deaths among users of tobacco or alcohol or both.

Although low-dose computed tomography in heavy current and former smokers has been shown to reduce lung cancer mortality and all-cause mortality in a clinical trial, the implementation of screening should proceed carefully to ensure that quality is high, best practices are met, and efforts are focused on reducing the high rate of false-positive findings. Meanwhile, tobacco control remains the most important global strategy for lung cancer control. There is little evidence to support population-based screening programs for cancers of the skin, stomach, and ovary, and the benefits of prostate specific antigen (PSA) testing may not outweigh the harms associated with over-diagnosis and overtreatment.

> "
> "To keep the body in good health is a duty...otherwise we shall not be able to keep our mind strong and clear."
>
> —Buddha

①
Screening programs vary between countries in how they are conducted.

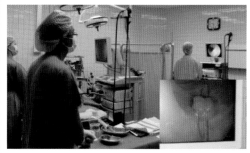

Colonoscopy in colorectal cancer screening program in Lampang, Thailand; a large bowel polyp is being removed during colonoscopy.

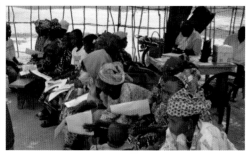

Women waiting for cervical screening using visual inspection with acetic acid in Conakry, Guinea.

②
In several high-income countries, cervical cancer incidence has shown a marked decrease with the advent of screening programs.

TRENDS IN CERVICAL CANCER AGE-STANDARDIZED INCIDENCE RATE (WORLD), 1953-2002

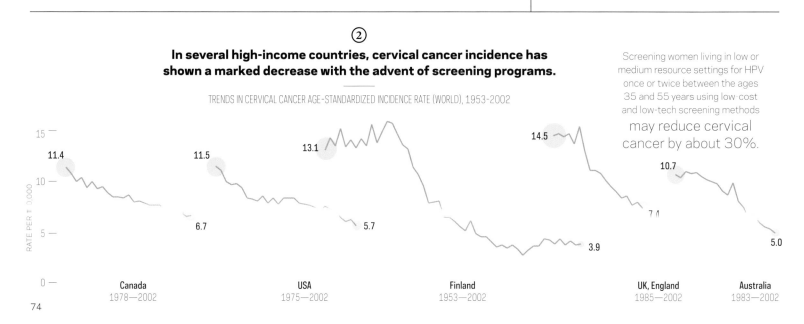

Screening women living in low or medium resource settings for HPV once or twice between the ages 35 and 55 years using low-cost and low-tech screening methods may reduce cervical cancer by about 30%.

RATE PER 100,000

15 —
10 —
5 —
0 —

11.4

11.5

13.1

14.5

10.7

6.7

5.7

7.4

3.9

5.0

Canada	USA	Finland	UK, England	Australia
1978—2002	1975—2002	1953—2002	1985—2002	1983—2002

Countries with large-scale colorectal screening programs
2014

Has a large-scale screening program

No large-scale screening program

A randomized clinical trial in the United Kingdom found that undergoing a single sigmoidoscopy **screening reduced colorectal cancer incidence and mortality by 33% and 43%, respectively.**

Countries with large-scale cervical and breast screening programs
2014

Cervical

Breast

No large-scale screening program

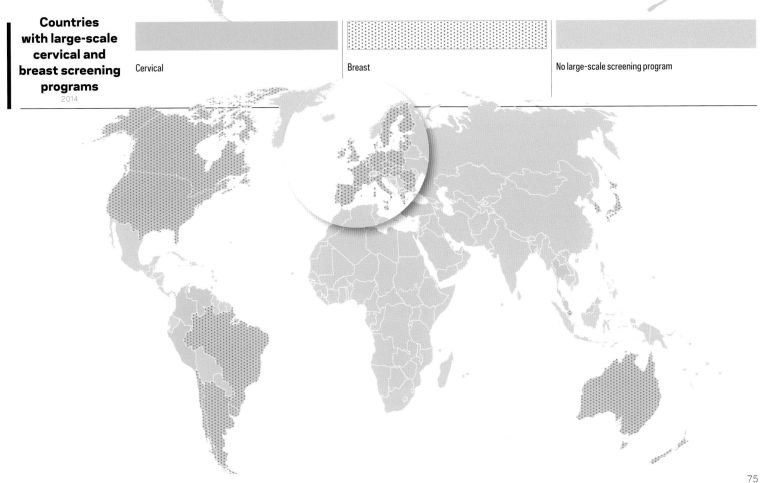

MANAGEMENT AND TREATMENT

Despite recent advances in cancer management and treatment, access to and cost of cancer care remain challenges in many countries.

①

The WHO List of Essential Medicines includes medicines associated with cancer survival increase at a relatively low cost that are also off-patent.

EXAMPLES OF MEDICINES FROM THE WHO ESSENTIAL MEDICINES LIST USED ALONE OR IN COMBINATION FOR CURATIVE TREATMENT OF COMMON CANCERS

BLEOMYCIN
(e.g. lymphomas and testicular cancers)

CALCIUM FOLINATE
(e.g. colorectal cancers)

CARBOPLATIN
(e.g. ovarian , testicular, lung , head and neck, bladder, and cervical cancers)

CHLORAMBUCIL
(e.g. chronic lymphocytic leukemia)

CYCLOPHOSPHAMIDE
(e.g. lymphomas, breast, and ovarian cancers)

CYTARABINE
(e.g. acute myeloblastic leukemia)

DOCETAXEL
(e.g. breast and ovarian cancers)

DOXORUBICIN
(e.g. breast, lymphomas, bladder, bone, and liver cancers)

ETOPOSIDE
(e.g. lymphomas, lung and testicular cancers)

FLUOROURACIL
(e.g. gastrointestinal tract and breast cancers)

IFOSFAMIDE
(e.g. bone sarcoma)

METHOTREXATE
(e.g. breast, bladder, leukemia, vesicular mole and sarcomas)

PACLITAXEL
(e.g. ovarian, breast, and lung cancers)

VINBLASTINE
(e.g. lymphomas, testicular and bladder cancers)

VINCRISTINE
(e.g. lymphomas and acute lymphocytic leukemia)

TAMOXIFEN
(e.g. breast cancer)

The primary modalities of cancer treatment are surgery, systemic therapy, and radiotherapy; these may be used alone or in combination. Of those cancer patients who are cured, curability is attributed as follows: surgery (49%), radiotherapy (40%) and chemotherapy (11%). Optimal treatment and diagnosis in early stages of disease have contributed to the decline in cancer mortality rates in most developed countries. In low- and middle-income countries (LMICs), limited access to affordable and quality cancer diagnosis and treatment has contributed to mortality-to-incidence ratios approximately 20% higher than those of industrialized countries.

The cost of cancer care has skyrocketed partly as a result of the development of expensive imaging techniques, radiation therapy equipment, and anticancer agents, including molecularly targeted therapies. As a result, the availability and receipt of treatment has been limited in many parts of the world. For example, despite approximately 60% of cancer patients being able to benefit at some point during the course of their disease from radiotherapy, this technology is far from being accessible to the 82% of the world's population living in the developing world. LMICs have 60% of new cancer cases but only 32% of the radiotherapy machines available worldwide. Africa and Southeast Asia face the largest shortages of radiotherapy units, with approximately 30 countries without radiotherapy services available.

Exacerbating the lack of access to modern diagnostic services, surgical oncology, radiotherapy equipment and chemotherapy is a drastic shortage of trained healthcare workers, which is a critical barrier to access to quality and equitable health services for cancer diagnosis and treatment. In Sub-Saharan Africa, trained pathologists, oncologists, and oncologic surgeons are exceedingly rare, and surgery is often performed by a general surgeon lacking specialty knowledge of cancer care. ③ Many countries in Sub-Saharan Africa average less than one pathologist per million population, and several lack even one trained medical oncologist or radiation oncologist.

Global scientific approaches and innovation are needed to ensure greater affordability of and access to better value cancer care for all. Policymakers and several organizations are currently working to expand patient access to therapy and increase the number of trained workforce personnel, although challenges in leveraging existing infrastructure and lowering costs remain.

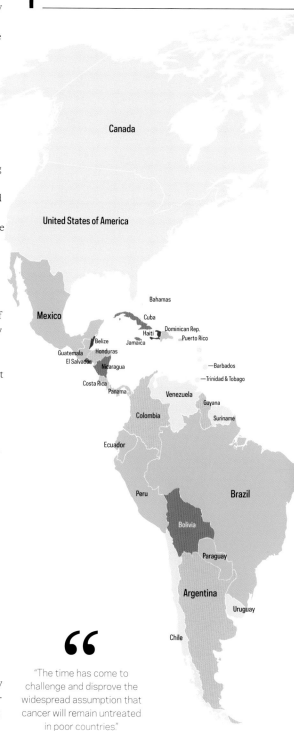

Estimation of radiotherapy coverage worldwide

PERCENTAGE OF PATIENTS NEEDING RADIOTHERAPY THAT CAN ACCESS THIS TREATMENT

"The time has come to challenge and disprove the widespread assumption that cancer will remain untreated in poor countries."

— Farmer P, et al. Lancet, 2010.

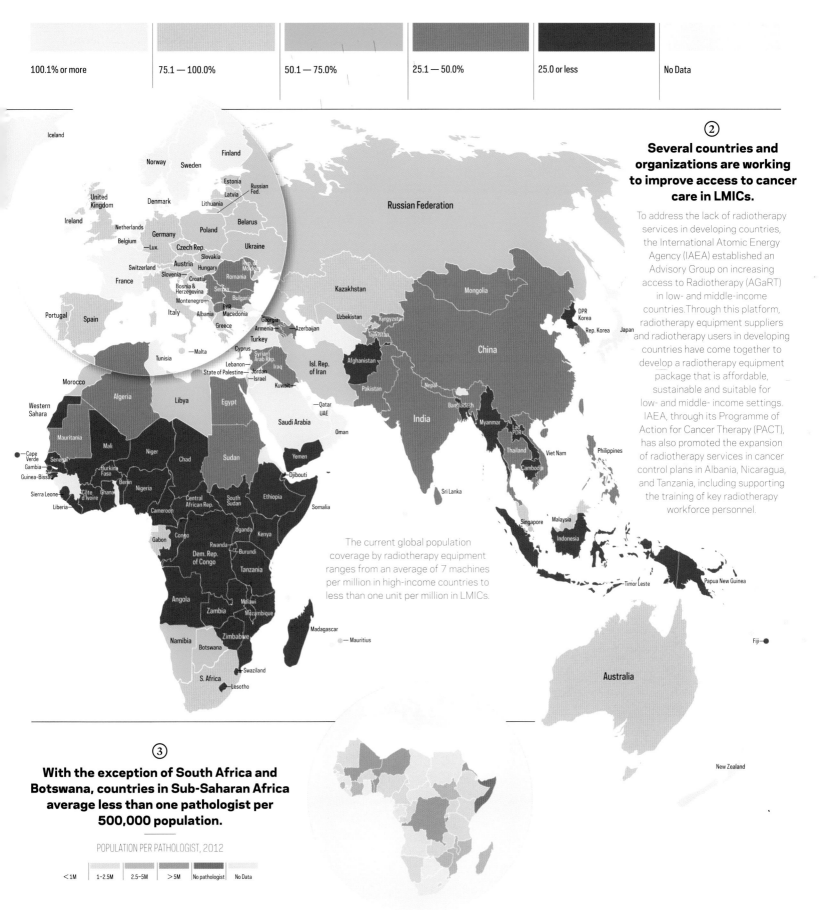

| 100.1% or more | 75.1 — 100.0% | 50.1 — 75.0% | 25.1 — 50.0% | 25.0 or less | No Data |

Iceland

Norway
Sweden
Finland

United
Kingdom
Denmark
Estonia
Latvia
Russian
Fed.
Lithuania

Ireland

Netherlands
Belgium
Lux.
Germany
Poland
Belarus
Ukraine

Switzerland
Austria
Czech Rep.
Slovakia
Hungary
Rep. of
Moldova
Romania

France
Slovenia
Croatia
Bosnia &
Herzegovina
Serbia
Bulgaria

Portugal
Spain
Italy
Montenegro
Albania
FYR
Macedonia

Greece

Malta

Tunisia

Cyprus
Syrian
Arab Rep.
Lebanon
State of Palestine
Jordan
Israel

Turkey
Georgia
Armenia
Azerbaijan

Iraq
Kuwait

Russian Federation

Kazakhstan

Mongolia

Uzbekistan
Kyrgyzstan
Tajikistan

DPR
Korea

Rep. Korea
Japan

Afghanistan
China

Morocco

Western
Sahara

Algeria
Libya
Egypt

Qatar
UAE
Saudi Arabia

Isl. Rep.
of Iran

Pakistan
Nepal

Oman

India
Bangladesh

Myanmar
Lao
PDR

Cape
Verde
Mauritania
Mali
Niger
Chad
Sudan
Yemen

Senegal
Gambia
Guinea-Bissau
Burkina
Faso
Benin
Nigeria

Sierra Leone
Côte
d'Ivoire
Ghana

Liberia

Cameroon
Central
African Rep.
South
Sudan
Ethiopia
Djibouti

Somalia

Thailand
Viet Nam
Philippines

Cambodia

Sri Lanka

Gabon
Congo
Uganda
Rwanda
Burundi
Kenya

Dem. Rep.
of Congo
Tanzania

Singapore
Malaysia

Indonesia

Angola
Malawi
Zambia
Mozambique

Madagascar
Mauritius

Timor Leste
Papua New Guinea

Namibia
Zimbabwe
Botswana

Swaziland
S. Africa
Lesotho

Fiji

Australia

New Zealand

② **Several countries and organizations are working to improve access to cancer care in LMICs.**

To address the lack of radiotherapy services in developing countries, the International Atomic Energy Agency (IAEA) established an Advisory Group on increasing access to Radiotherapy (AGaRT) in low- and middle-income countries. Through this platform, radiotherapy equipment suppliers and radiotherapy users in developing countries have come together to develop a radiotherapy equipment package that is affordable, sustainable and suitable for low- and middle- income settings. IAEA, through its Programme of Action for Cancer Therapy (PACT), has also promoted the expansion of radiotherapy services in cancer control plans in Albania, Nicaragua, and Tanzania, including supporting the training of key radiotherapy workforce personnel.

The current global population coverage by radiotherapy equipment ranges from an average of 7 machines per million in high-income countries to less than one unit per million in LMICs.

③ **With the exception of South Africa and Botswana, countries in Sub-Saharan Africa average less than one pathologist per 500,000 population.**

POPULATION PER PATHOLOGIST, 2012

| < 1M | 1-2.5M | 2.5-5M | > 5M | No pathologist | No Data |

PAIN CONTROL

Access to opioid analgesics for pain relief is severely limited in most low- and middle-income countries.

Opioid analgesics, including morphine, are considered essential medicines by the World Health Organization and are recommended for the treatment of moderate to severe pain.

① Opioids are also on almost all national essential medicines lists, but access to them is severely limited in most low- and middle-income countries, where 85% of the world's population consumes just 7% of the medicinal opioids.

② There is no more striking example of the global disparity in access to health care than pain relief in cancer.

Approximately 80% of people with advanced cancer experience moderate to severe pain. Untreated pain that grows worse each day is a consistent feature of cancer care in most resource-limited settings.

Although morphine, the most effective treatment for severe pain, is safe, effective, plentiful, inexpensive, and easy to use, legal and regulatory restrictions, cultural misperceptions about pain, inadequate training of healthcare providers, a poorly functioning market, generally weak health systems, and concern about diversion, addiction, and abuse create a web of barriers that force millions of people to live and die with treatable pain.

The provision of pain relief is the mandate of national governments, and several governments are taking steps to improve access to pain relief. In particular, Nigeria, which is home to approximately 20% of the population of Sub-Saharan Africa, has embarked on a new initiative to improve access to oral morphine. The government of Uganda now makes oral morphine available to patients at no cost, and the government of Kenya has committed to expanding availability of pain relief through the public sector.

①

Access to pain relief is strongly correlated with country income level.

NUMBER OF DEATHS IN PAIN, 2011

Deaths in pain due to cancer or HIV

Treated deaths in pain

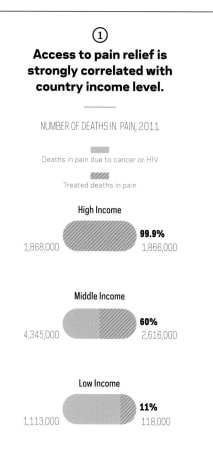

High Income
1,868,000 — 99.9% — 1,866,000

Middle Income
4,345,000 — 60% — 2,616,000

Low Income
1,113,000 — 11% — 118,000

②

Sub-Saharan Africa & South Asia are home to 73% of the world's untreated deaths in pain.

PERCENTAGE OF DEATHS THAT ARE NOT TREATED FOR PAIN BY REGION, 2011

Europe & Central Asia **8%**

Latin America & Caribbean **4%**

East Asia & Pacific **12%**

South Asia **31%**

Sub-Saharan Africa **43%**

Untreated deaths in pain
2011

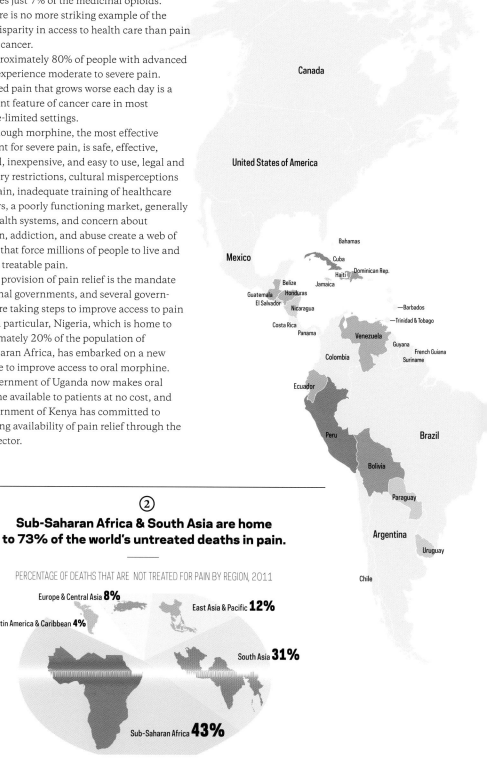

Canada

United States of America

Mexico

Bahamas

Cuba

Haiti

Dominican Rep.

Belize

Jamaica

Guatemala
El Salvador

Honduras

Nicaragua

Barbados

Trinidad & Tobago

Costa Rica

Panama

Venezuela

Guyana

French Guiana

Suriname

Colombia

Ecuador

Peru

Brazil

Bolivia

Paraguay

Argentina

Uruguay

Chile

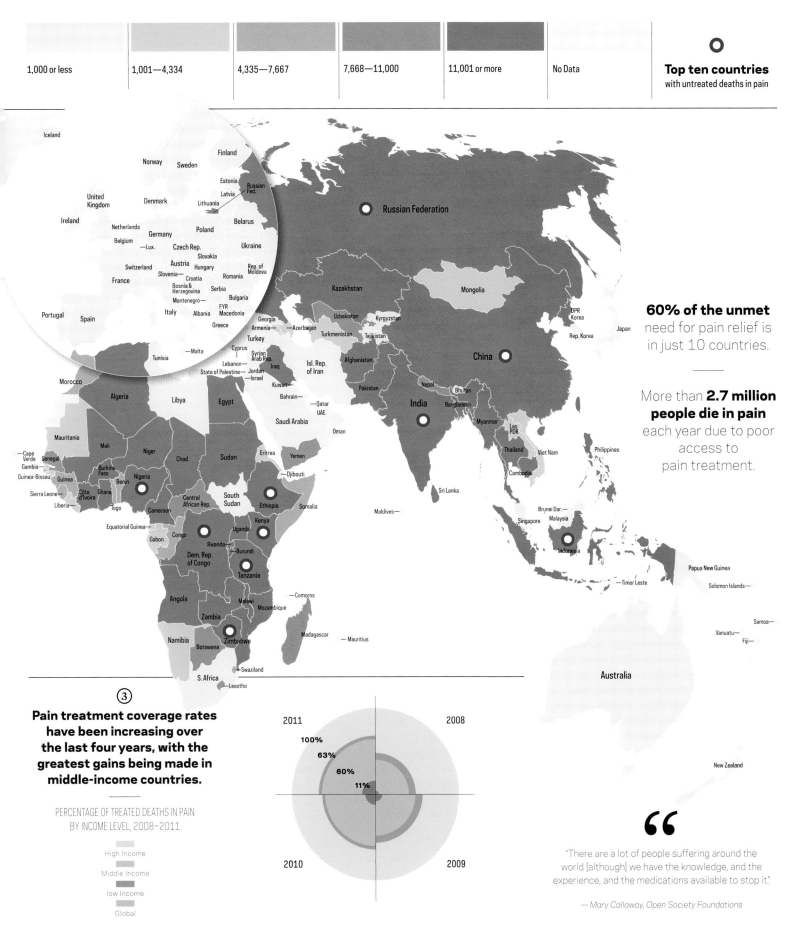

| 1,000 or less | 1,001—4,334 | 4,335—7,667 | 7,668—11,000 | 11,001 or more | No Data |

Top ten countries
with untreated deaths in pain

60% of the unmet need for pain relief is in just 10 countries.

More than **2.7 million people die in pain** each year due to poor access to pain treatment.

③

Pain treatment coverage rates have been increasing over the last four years, with the greatest gains being made in middle-income countries.

PERCENTAGE OF TREATED DEATHS IN PAIN
BY INCOME LEVEL, 2008–2011

High Income
Middle Income
low Income
Global

2011   2008
100%
63%
60%
11%

2010   2009

"There are a lot of people suffering around the world [although] we have the knowledge, and the experience, and the medications available to stop it."

— Mary Callaway, Open Society Foundations

CANCER REGISTRIES

The Surveillance of Cancer:

Reliable cancer incidence and mortality data are an ever-growing need, particularly in low- and medium-Human Development Index settings.

The reliable monitoring and surveillance of cancer is essential for the development of cancer control plans. Cancer registries fulfill this requirement by collecting cancer incidence data for defined populations, including information on patient and tumor characteristics at diagnosis (e.g. patient age, tumor type), and in some cases stage at diagnosis, type of treatment received, and outcome. Population-based cancer registries may cover an entire national population or a smaller region within a country, such as a province or county. Registry quality varies widely by geographic region; many countries in Latin America, Asia and Africa have poor quality or a complete absence of incidence data.

Population-based cancer registries throughout the world are represented by the International Association of Cancer Registries (IACR) (*http://www.iacr.com.fr/*), an organization founded in 1966 that provides opportunities for cancer registry personnel to meet, exchange information, and receive training. Approximately every five years, IACR collaborates with the International Agency for Research on Cancer (IARC) to publish *Cancer Incidence in Five Continents* (CI5) (*http://ci5.iarc.fr*), which contains cancer incidence data from the highest-quality registries worldwide. These registries represent a major source of information for GLOBOCAN

(*http://globocan.iarc.fr*), a summary of estimated cancer statistics from which most of the cancer maps in *The Cancer Atlas* are derived. In countries where no cancer registry data are available, or only very limited information from case series, incidence must be approximated from mortality information (where available) or from incidence in neighboring countries.

① Although there are significant disparities in cancer registry development, the number of high-quality cancer registries published in CI5 is increasing. Volume I, covering the early 1960s, had data from 31 cancer registries in 28 countries. The most recent volume (Volume X), covering 2003-07, has data from 290 registries in 68 countries. The multi-agency Global Initiative for Cancer Registry Development (*http://gicr.iarc.fr*) aims to bring about quantum changes in the availability of high-quality cancer registry data in these regions within the next decade.

② Cancer death (or vital) registration data are also important for planning and monitoring cancer control programs. As with cancer registry data, there is wide international variation in the quality and completeness of death certificate information, with many countries in low- and medium-Human Development Index regions having poor quality or a complete absence of vital registration.

---

① **Cancer registry inclusion and population coverage in *Cancer Incidence in Five Continents* has grown exponentially since the first volume.**

② **In many parts of the world, such as Latin America, Africa, and Asia, high-quality cancer incidence and mortality data are extremely lacking.**

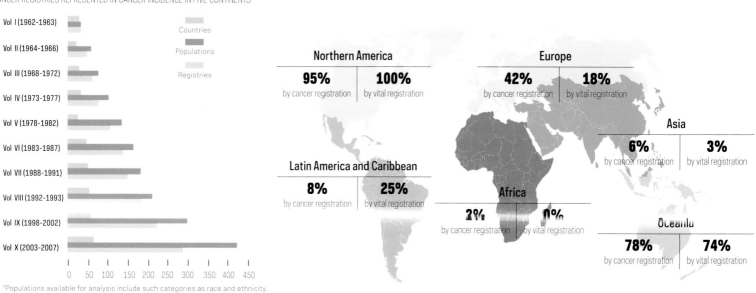

NUMBER OF COUNTRIES, POPULATIONS AVAILABLE FOR ANALYSIS,* AND CANCER REGISTRIES REPRESENTED IN *CANCER INCIDENCE IN FIVE CONTINENTS*

Vol I (1962-1963)
Vol II (1964-1966)
Vol III (1968-1972)
Vol IV (1973-1977)
Vol V (1978-1982)
Vol VI (1983-1987)
Vol VII (1988-1991)
Vol VIII (1992-1993)
Vol IX (1998-2002)
Vol X (2003-2007)

Countries
Populations
Registries

0 50 100 150 200 250 300 350 400 450

*Populations available for analysis include such categories as race and ethnicity.

PROPORTION (%) OF THE REGIONAL POPULATION COVERED BY HIGH-QUALITY CANCER REGISTRATION AND HIGH-QUALITY COMPLETE VITAL REGISTRATION OF DEATH

HIGHEST HDI REGION ← → LOWEST HDI REGION

Northern America
95% by cancer registration | **100%** by vital registration

Europe
42% by cancer registration | **18%** by vital registration

Asia
6% by cancer registration | **3%** by vital registration

Latin America and Caribbean
8% by cancer registration | **25%** by vital registration

Africa
2% by cancer registration | **0%** by vital registration

Oceania
78% by cancer registration | **74%** by vital registration

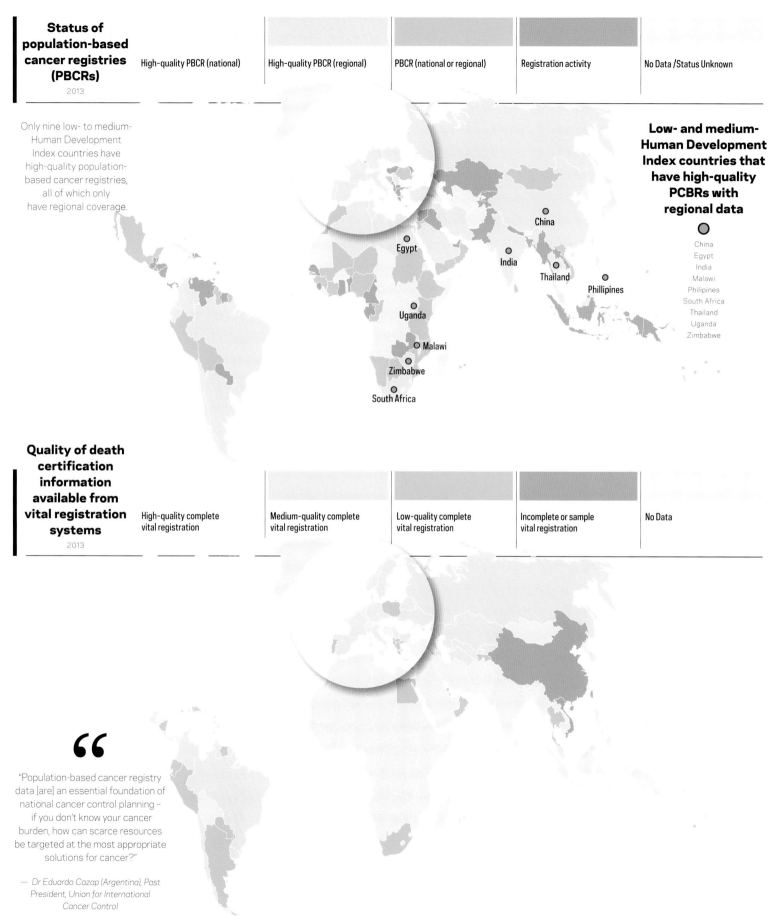

Status of population-based cancer registries (PBCRs)
2013

High-quality PBCR (national)	High-quality PBCR (regional)	PBCR (national or regional)	Registration activity	No Data /Status Unknown

Only nine low- to medium-Human Development Index countries have high-quality population-based cancer registries, all of which only have regional coverage.

Low- and medium-Human Development Index countries that have high-quality PCBRs with regional data

China
Egypt
India
Malawi
Philipines
South Africa
Thailand
Uganda
Zimbabwe

China
Egypt
India
Thailand
Phillipines
Uganda
Malawi
Zimbabwe
South Africa

Quality of death certification information available from vital registration systems
2013

High-quality complete vital registration	Medium-quality complete vital registration	Low-quality complete vital registration	Incomplete or sample vital registration	No Data

"

"Population-based cancer registry data [are] an essential foundation of national cancer control planning – if you don't know your cancer burden, how can scarce resources be targeted at the most appropriate solutions for cancer?"

— Dr Eduardo Cazap (Argentina), Past President, Union for International Cancer Control

RESEARCH

Medicines and fundamental biology dominate cancer research in high-income countries.

Cancer research spans all disciplines of science, from the social and humanistic to fundamental biomedicine. ① Cancer research in wealthy countries dominates disease-specific biomedical research. ② However, most research funding is skewed towards fundamental biology and treatment, particularly cancer medicines. While this has delivered an impressive amount of knowledge as well as new medicines and biomarkers, many parts of the world and areas of cancer research have been left behind. For example, prevention research attracts less than 5% of funding. Global cancer is challenged by a wide variety of issues, including sustainability, disincentives for research for the public good rather than for commercial benefit, and mismatch between funding and research need.

Only a fraction (2.7%) of global investment in cancer research is spent on research directly relevant to low- and middle-income countries. Rather than development of new innovative technologies or drugs, there must be greater focus on optimizing utilization of available drugs and radiation technologies in cost-effective ways that meet the needs of low- and middle-income countries. ③ Orphan domains of research, such as prevention and cancer surgery, also need to be addressed.

Implementation research, which seeks to apply new scientific research findings, is another neglected area in global cancer research. This gap between development of scientific discoveries in cancer and their actual use to improve outcomes for patients emphasizes the need for more independent, publicly-funded research to be dedicated to solving research questions that have high public good, but low commercial attraction, for example in global childhood cancers and cost-effective screening.

④ There is also increasing global recognition that a national-level research is essential; for example, many countries in the Middle East and North Africa have begun to substantially engage in the cancer research agenda. However, global research remains far too exclusively centered in high-income countries.

How can we promote and drive equity in global cancer research in low- and middle-income countries? Twinning partnerships between high-income and low- and middle-income centers have already proved effective and could be expanded. A global cancer fund would provide much-needed resources to link networks and centers to build capacity and research; training and education in research methodologies always produces results. But ultimately, more research funding must be directed at global cancer research partnerships, and national cancer research capability needs to be built, particularly focused on orphan areas such as surgery.

①

Cancer research papers are dominated by the highest Human Development Index countries

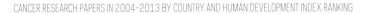

CANCER RESEARCH PAPERS IN 2004-2013 BY COUNTRY AND HUMAN DEVELOPMENT INDEX RANKING

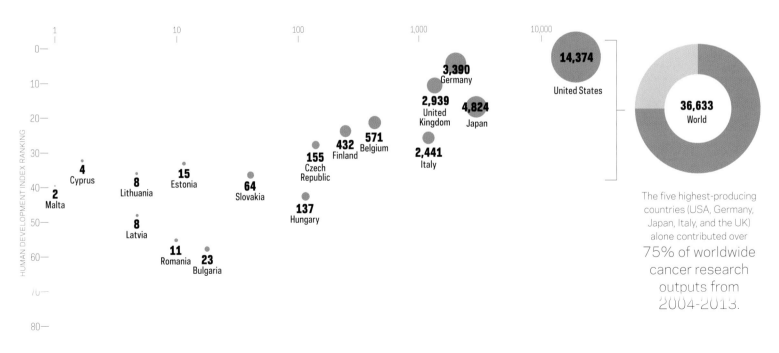

The five highest-producing countries (USA, Germany, Japan, Italy, and the UK) alone contributed over 75% of worldwide cancer research outputs from 2004-2013.

② The majority of cancer research funding continues to go towards understanding the biology and treatment of cancer.

PERCENTAGE OF CANCER RESEARCH FUNDING
ALLOCATED BY COMMON SCIENTIFIC OUTLINE CATEGORY IN EUROPE, 2002-2003

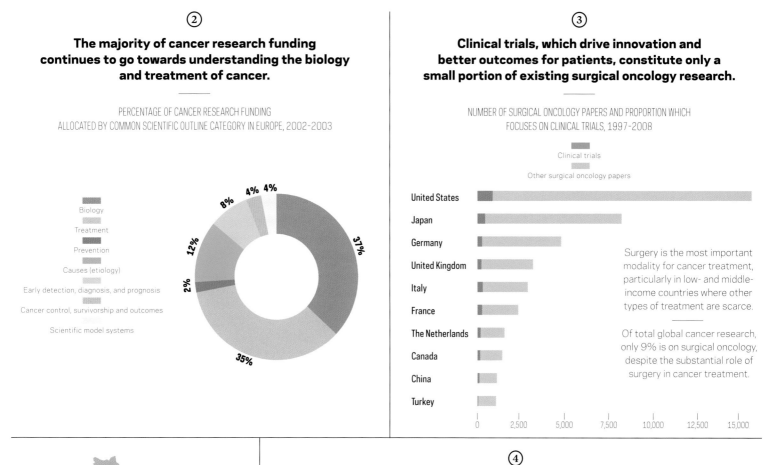

- Biology
- Treatment
- Prevention
- Causes (etiology)
- Early detection, diagnosis, and prognosis
- Cancer control, survivorship and outcomes
- Scientific model systems

37% · 35% · 2% · 12% · 8% · 4% · 4%

③ Clinical trials, which drive innovation and better outcomes for patients, constitute only a small portion of existing surgical oncology research.

NUMBER OF SURGICAL ONCOLOGY PAPERS AND PROPORTION WHICH
FOCUSES ON CLINICAL TRIALS, 1997-2008

- Clinical trials
- Other surgical oncology papers

United States, Japan, Germany, United Kingdom, Italy, France, The Netherlands, Canada, China, Turkey

0 · 2,500 · 5,000 · 7,500 · 10,000 · 12,500 · 15,000

Surgery is the most important modality for cancer treatment, particularly in low- and middle-income countries where other types of treatment are scarce.

Of total global cancer research, only 9% is on surgical oncology, despite the substantial role of surgery in cancer treatment.

India has now developed a partnership of 52 cancer centers (National Cancer Grid) dedicated to driving care quality and research across all states.

"In the temple of science are many mansions, and various indeed are they that dwell therein."
— Albert Einstein

④ Although cancer research continues to occur predominantly in high-income countries, many countries in the Middle East and North Africa have begun to substantially engage in the cancer research agenda.

NUMBER OF CANCER RESEARCH PAPERS AND PERCENTAGE OF INTERNATIONAL COLLABORATIONS IN THE MIDDLE EAST OVER THE LAST TEN YEARS

- Percentage of cancer research co-authored with international collaborators

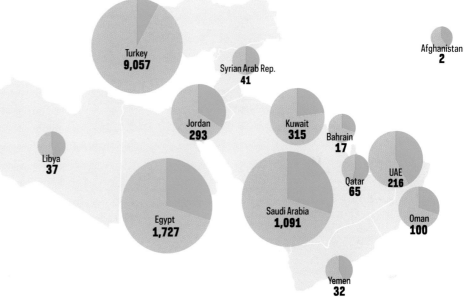

Turkey 9,057 · Syrian Arab Rep. 41 · Afghanistan 2 · Jordan 293 · Kuwait 315 · Bahrain 17 · Libya 37 · Qatar 65 · UAE 216 · Egypt 1,727 · Saudi Arabia 1,091 · Oman 100 · Yemen 32

INVESTING IN CANCER PREVENTION

Population-based measures can prevent cancer at a low cost.

International aid for cancer prevention and control in the world's poorest nations is miniscule. Resources to fight all non-communicable diseases, including cancer, plunged during the global economic crisis, and amounted to a mere 1.2% of the total development assistance for health in 2011.

(2)
Investing in cancer prevention not only saves lives, but the money saved could also pay for important services and institutions.

Facing scarce resources, policymakers must determine how best to invest in their country's future. Investment in health can save costs and facilitate economic growth by increasing productivity. Economic analyses help governments and international donors identify health practices that are not only feasible, but also the best value for money.

(1) The exact global cost of cancer is unknown, but it is undoubtedly well into the hundreds of billions of dollars per year. In the United States alone, the estimated cost of cancer in 2009, including direct medical costs as well as the cost of lost productivity due to premature death, was US$216.6 billion per year. The global cost of cancer is expected to increase due to increases in the number of new cancer cases as well as the growing cost of cancer therapies.

(2) However, a substantial part of this cost can be averted by investing in cancer prevention, early detection, and treatment (see chapter 24—*The Cancer Continuum*). For example, cost-effective strategies to address common cancer risk factors such as tobacco use, alcohol abuse, unhealthy diet and physical inactivity in low- and middle-income countries would cost only US$2 billion per year, a small amount compared to the costs incurred by the total disease burden. (3) (4) For example, in developing countries, cervical cancer screenings that require little laboratory infrastructure, such as simple visual inspection of the cervix with acetic acid or DNA testing for HPV in cervical cell samples, cost less than US$500 per year of life saved. In general, cancer prevention is far more cost-effective than treatment.

(1)
The total cost of cancer in the European Union is more than the entire EU budget.

IN BILLION (BN) EUROS IN 2009

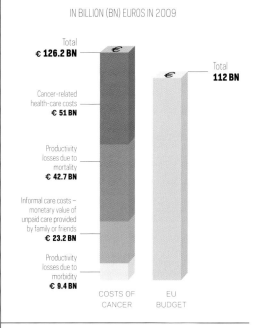

Total
€ 126.2 BN

Cancer-related health-care costs
€ 51 BN

Productivity losses due to mortality
€ 42.7 BN

Informal care costs – monetary value of unpaid care provided by family or friends
€ 23.2 BN

Productivity losses due to morbidity
€ 9.4 BN

Total
112 BN

COSTS OF CANCER   EU BUDGET

"
"It is health that is real wealth, and not pieces of gold and silver."

— *Mahatma Gandhi*

U.S.
Intervention
COLORECTAL SCREENING
Colonoscopy in population of 50 to 64 year olds

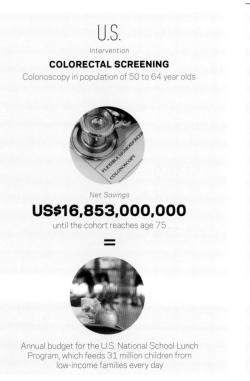

Net Savings
US$16,853,000,000
until the cohort reaches age 75

=

Annual budget for the U.S. National School Lunch Program, which feeds 31 million children from low-income families every day

TAIPEI, CHINA
Intervention
SMOKING CESSATION SERVICES PROGRAM
Counseling and nicotine replacement therapy

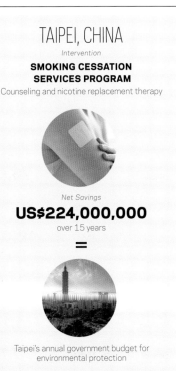

Net Savings
US$224,000,000
over 15 years

=

Taipei's annual government budget for environmental protection

AUSTRALIA
Intervention
THE AUSTRALIAN NATIONAL TOBACCO CAMPAIGN
An intensive 6-month mass media anti-smoking campaign

Net Savings
US$912,000,000
over the remaining lifetime of the 190,000 quitters

=

Australia's governmental investment in early childhood education

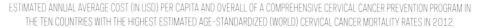

③

Cervical cancer prevention programs are very affordable.

ESTIMATED ANNUAL AVERAGE COST (IN USD) PER CAPITA AND OVERALL OF A COMPREHENSIVE CERVICAL CANCER PREVENTION PROGRAM IN THE TEN COUNTRIES WITH THE HIGHEST ESTIMATED AGE-STANDARDIZED (WORLD) CERVICAL CANCER MORTALITY RATES IN 2012.

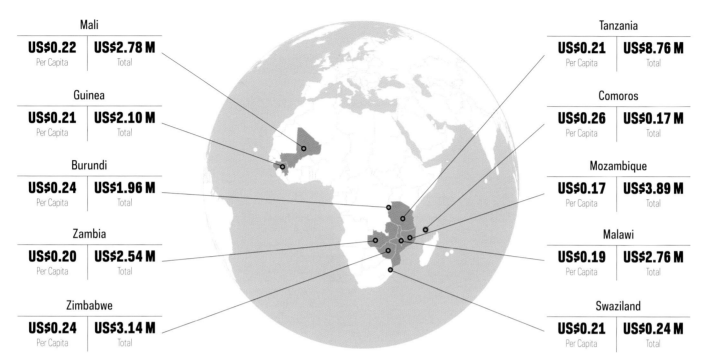

Mali
US$0.22	US$2.78 M
Per Capita	Total

Guinea
US$0.21	US$2.10 M
Per Capita	Total

Burundi
US$0.24	US$1.96 M
Per Capita	Total

Zambia
US$0.20	US$2.54 M
Per Capita	Total

Zimbabwe
US$0.24	US$3.14 M
Per Capita	Total

Tanzania
US$0.21	US$8.76 M
Per Capita	Total

Comoros
US$0.26	US$0.17 M
Per Capita	Total

Mozambique
US$0.17	US$3.89 M
Per Capita	Total

Malawi
US$0.19	US$2.76 M
Per Capita	Total

Swaziland
US$0.21	US$0.24 M
Per Capita	Total

These estimated costs cover primary care outpatient visits for consultation, counseling and procedures, auxiliary care, medicines, and diagnostic and therapeutic procedures.

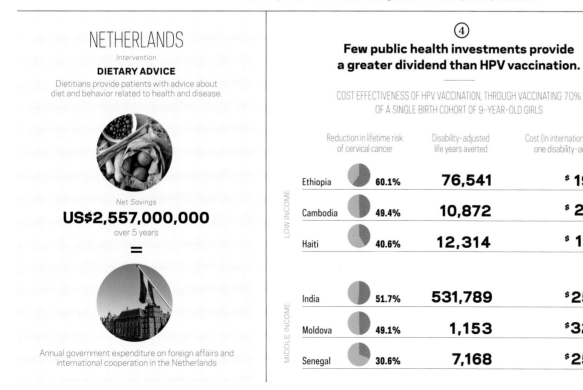

NETHERLANDS
Intervention
DIETARY ADVICE
Dietitians provide patients with advice about diet and behavior related to health and disease.

Net Savings
US$2,557,000,000
over 5 years

=

Annual government expenditure on foreign affairs and international cooperation in the Netherlands

④

Few public health investments provide a greater dividend than HPV vaccination.

COST EFFECTIVENESS OF HPV VACCINATION, THROUGH VACCINATING 70% OF A SINGLE BIRTH COHORT OF 9-YEAR-OLD GIRLS

	Reduction in lifetime risk of cervical cancer	Disability-adjusted life years averted	Cost (in international dollars) to avert one disability-adjusted life year
LOW INCOME			
Ethiopia	60.1%	76,541	$ 190
Cambodia	49.4%	10,872	$ 210
Haiti	40.6%	12,314	$ 110
MIDDLE INCOME			
India	51.7%	531,789	$ 250
Moldova	49.1%	1,153	$ 320
Senegal	30.6%	7,168	$ 250

At a price negotiated by GAVI of approximately US $5 per dose, HPV vaccination of preadolescent girls will cost less than gross domestic product per capita for one disability-adjusted life year averted, which by WHO standards makes the vaccination intervention very cost-effective.

LEVERAGING EXISTING INFRASTRUCTURE

Resources for cancer prevention and control are severely limited in many low- and middle-income countries, but existing public health workforce and infrastructure can be leveraged across infectious and chronic diseases to increase their impact.

Leveraging existing public health infrastructure is an important strategy for cancer control in low- and middle-income countries, where resources to address the burden of chronic disease are limited. Building public health capacity in developing countries has historically stemmed from efforts to combat infectious diseases—responses to HIV/AIDS, tuberculosis, malaria, and natural disasters have strengthened the infrastructure and work-force for health and laboratory services, disease surveillance, and public health training programs.

(1) The United States Centers for Disease Control and Prevention (CDC) works with ministries of health and other partners to establish sustainable Field Epidemiology Training Programs (FETPs), which help to build and strengthen workforce capacity for disease detection, laboratory services, and outbreak response. Since 1980, 50 of these programs have produced more than 2,800 graduates in 69 countries, with more than 80% of graduates serving as public health leaders in their home countries. There is great potential to leverage FETP infrastructure and expertise to build capacity and leadership for the prevention and control of cancer and other chronic diseases.

Established in 2003 in response to the AIDS pandemic, the United States President's Emergency Plan for AIDS Relief (PEPFAR) has enabled the development of an increasingly important platform for the control of a number of diseases, including cervical and breast cancer — PEPFAR-facilitated infrastructure has served as a springboard for women's cancer initiatives in more than 15 countries. (2) Among these is the Pink Ribbon Red Ribbon (PRRR) initiative, an innovative public-private partnership that uses evidence-based approaches to deliver healthcare services for women's cancers. PRRR-supported programs increase access to cervical cancer screening and treatment, human papillomavirus (HPV) vaccine, and breast and cervical cancer education for underserved women.

(3) There are many opportunities to leverage existing public health workforce and infrastructure across infectious and chronic diseases. Amidst an increasing burden of cancer and limited funding for cancer programs, this strategy can increase the impact of resources devoted to cancer prevention and control in low- and middle-income countries.

"

"Poor people endure a double burden of communicable and non-communicable chronic illness, requiring a response that is well integrated into the health systems of low-income and middle-income countries. Extension of cancer prevention, diagnosis, and treatment to millions of people with or at risk of cancer is an urgent health and ethical priority."

— Farmer P, et al.
Lancet 2010.

(1) CDC-supported Field Epidemiology Training Programs (FETPs)

Since 1980,
50 CDC-supported FETPs have produced more than 2,800 graduates in 69 countries
(not including the US Epidemiologic Intelligence Service).

In 2011, CDC developed open access training materials in chronic disease epidemiology, which were piloted in 6 FETP focus countries.

CDC and the US National Cancer Institute are currently developing a cancer curriculum for low-resource settings.

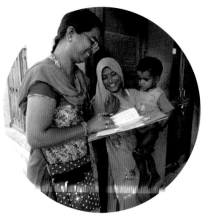

India Epidemic Intelligence Service Officer conducting an immunization coverage survey in Rajasthan, India.

(2) Pink Ribbon Red Ribbon (PRRR)

Since 2011, more than 250 healthcare providers at PRRR-supported sites in Sub-Saharan Africa have been trained in the "see and treat" approach to cervical cancer screening.
More than 5,000 women have been screened for breast cancer in Tanzania.

More than 100,000 women have been screened
for cervical cancer at PRRR-supported sites in Botswana, Zambia, and Tanzania.

Nearly 19,000 girls
have received the full three doses of the HPV vaccine through PRRR-supported vaccine demonstration programs.

Field Epidemiology Training Programs (FETPs)

2014

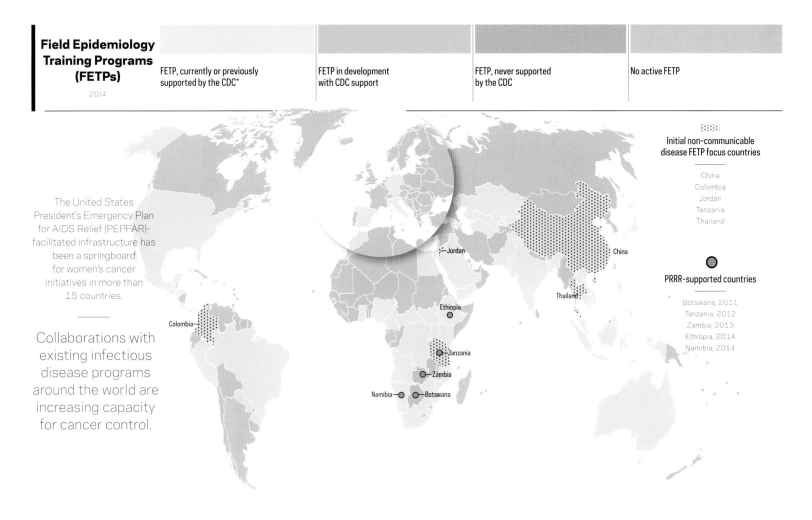

| FETP, currently or previously supported by the CDC* | FETP in development with CDC support | FETP, never supported by the CDC | No active FETP |

The United States President's Emergency Plan for AIDS Relief (PEPFAR)-facilitated infrastructure has been a springboard for women's cancer initiatives in more than 15 countries.

Collaborations with existing infectious disease programs around the world are increasing capacity for cancer control.

Colombia

Jordan

China

Thailand

Ethiopia

Tanzania

Zambia

Namibia — Botswana

Initial non-communicable disease FETP focus countries

China
Colombia
Jordan
Tanzania
Thailand

PRRR-supported countries

Botswana, 2011
Tanzania, 2012
Zambia, 2013
Ethiopia, 2014
Namibia, 2014

*The training program in the USA refers to the CDC's Epidemiologic Intelligence Service

---

(3)
World Health Organization (WHO)

The GAVI Alliance has worked with the WHO Expanded Program on Immunization (EPI) to prevent cervical and liver cancers in low-income countries by increasing access to HPV and hepatitis B vaccines.

The WHO list of essential medications and its prequalification program for manufacturers of antiretroviral drugs for HIV/AIDS can be used to increase access to generic drugs for chemotherapy and palliative care in low- and middle-income countries.

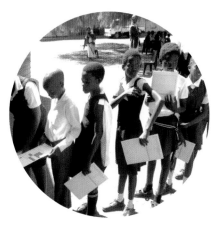

School girls in Botswana awaiting HPV vaccination.

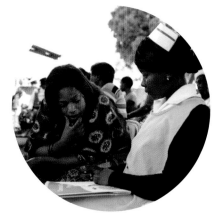

Healthcare worker explains cervical cancer screening and treatment process, Mosi-Oa-Tunya Clinic, Livingstone, Zambia.

UNITING ORGANIZATIONS

We have the tools and know-how to improve survival and quality of life; a cancer community united behind comprehensive cancer plans will harness the political drive for real national impact by 2025.

①

Creative opportunities exist to convene stakeholders within and beyond the cancer community.

World Cancer Leaders' Summit

This annual high-level policy meeting is an opportunity to reach key decision-makers, and to identify new and innovative solutions with thought-leaders in the cancer field.

uicc
global cancer control
WORLD CANCER CONGRESS

The biennial World Cancer Congress provides a forum for cancer control experts, practitioners, and advocates to share the latest information on global advances in cancer control.

World Cancer Day (February 4) is the single initiative which unites the entire world in the global fight against cancer, raising general awareness around the disease.

The cancer community—including cancer societies, research and treatment centers, patient support groups, and survivors at the local, national and global levels—is engaged in a broad spectrum of activity from fundraising, research, advocacy, and health education to cancer surveillance, treatment and care. ① Many cancer-related issues require solutions outside of health; developing synergistic partnerships across sectors (education, labor, finance, and development) and with key stakeholders (government, United Nations agencies, civil society organizations, and the private sector where appropriate) is critical to accelerating progress in cancer prevention and control.

In support of this goal, the World Cancer Declaration unites the cancer community behind a set of global visionary targets and priority actions—many of which are now embedded in global commitments on non-communicable diseases. The World Cancer Declaration calls upon government leaders and health policy-makers to significantly reduce the global cancer burden, promote greater equity, and integrate cancer control into the world health and development agenda. Innovative and strategic multi-sectorial partnerships like the following are fundamental to delivering the targets of the World Cancer Declaration and achieving the global target of reducing premature deaths from non-communicable diseases (NCDs) by 25% by 2025:

INTERNATIONAL CANCER CONTROL PARTNERSHIP (ICCP)
is helping governments to develop and implement effective national cancer control plans.
www.iccp-portal.org

FRAMEWORK CONVENTION ALLIANCE (FCA)
is supporting global tobacco control efforts through the World Health Organization (WHO) Framework Convention on Tobacco Control.
www.fctc.org

GLOBAL TASKFORCE ON RADIOTHERAPY FOR CANCER CONTROL
is working to identify the investment needed to provide equity in global access to radiation therapy.
www.uicc.org/advocacy/our-campaigns/global-task-force-radiotherapy-cancer-control

GLOBAL INITIATIVE FOR CANCER REGISTRY DEVELOPMENT
is working to develop and build registry capacity worldwide.
http://gicr.iarc.fr/

REACH TO RECOVERY INTERNATIONAL
improves the quality of life for women with breast cancer and their families through peer support and advocacy.
www.reachtorecoveryinternational.org

THE MCCABE CENTRE FOR LAW AND CANCER
is building capacity for the effective use of law in cancer control.
www.mccabecentre.org

THE NCD ALLIANCE, unites over 2,000 civil society organizations to raise the profile of NCDs as a development priority.
www.ncdalliance.org

A palliative care advocacy network that includes the **UNION FOR INTERNATIONAL CANCER CONTROL, HUMAN RIGHTS WATCH,** and the **WORLD PALLIATIVE CARE ASSOCIATION** is working together to position palliative care on the WHO agenda and drive action at a national level.

A global network of cancer-fighting organizations
ORGANIZATIONS PER COUNTRY

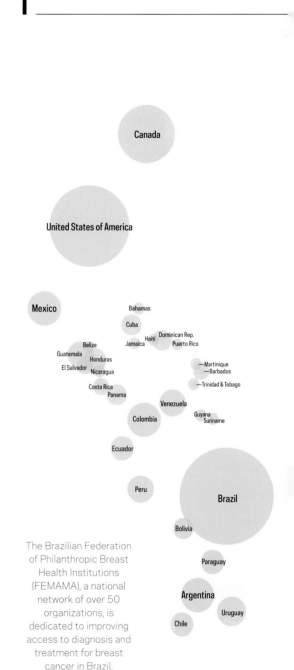

The Brazilian Federation of Philanthropic Breast Health Institutions (FEMAMA), a national network of over 50 organizations, is dedicated to improving access to diagnosis and treatment for breast cancer in Brazil.

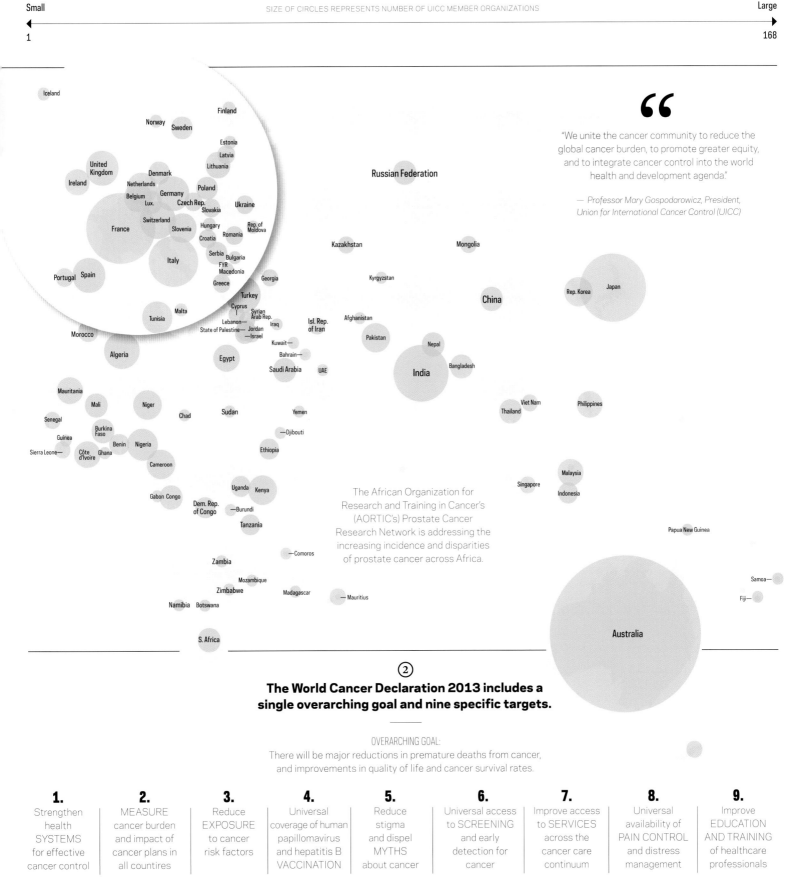

"We unite the cancer community to reduce the global cancer burden, to promote greater equity, and to integrate cancer control into the world health and development agenda."

— Professor Mary Gospodarowicz, President, Union for International Cancer Control (UICC)

The African Organization for Research and Training in Cancer's (AORTIC's) Prostate Cancer Research Network is addressing the increasing incidence and disparities of prostate cancer across Africa.

②

The World Cancer Declaration 2013 includes a single overarching goal and nine specific targets.

OVERARCHING GOAL:
There will be major reductions in premature deaths from cancer, and improvements in quality of life and cancer survival rates.

1.	2.	3.	4.	5.	6.	7.	8.	9.
Strengthen health SYSTEMS for effective cancer control	MEASURE cancer burden and impact of cancer plans in all countires	Reduce EXPOSURE to cancer risk factors	Universal coverage of human papillomavirus and hepatitis B VACCINATION	Reduce stigma and dispel MYTHS about cancer	Universal access to SCREENING and early detection for cancer	Improve access to SERVICES across the cancer care continuum	Universal availability of PAIN CONTROL and distress management	Improve EDUCATION AND TRAINING of healthcare professionals

GLOBAL RELAY FOR LIFE

Global Relay For Life celebrates survivors, remembers loved ones lost, and fights back against cancer.

> **"**
> "All communities which have participated in Relay For Life have seen the change it is making in their communities. In every community where a Relay is taking place, a light of hope has been lit."
>
> — Sandra Jacobs, Volunteer, Cancer Association of South Africa

Since its beginnings with one man in Tacoma, USA in 1985, the American Cancer Society Relay For Life program has turned into a global movement spanning all continents, giving a voice to cancer survivors and caregivers, and mobilizing people to take up the fight against cancer. (1) Today, Relay raises nearly USD 500 million annually engaging 24 countries in the fight. (2) Relay is now the largest fund-raising movement in the world, raising over USD 5 billion since its founding.

Global Relay For Life provides an opportunity for participants to celebrate survivors, remember loved ones lost, and fight back against a disease that takes too many. More than a fundraiser, Relay For Life fosters hope, healing, and inspiration in over 6,000 communities across the world.

Global Relay For Life empowers local cancer organizations to promote community cancer awareness, advocate for change, and reduce the burden of this disease. Relay volunteers globally have advocated for change, sending tens of thousands of petitions to Parliament in Australia to pass their largest colorectal cancer screening bill in history, while survivors from Jamaica and the United Kingdom brought their voices to the United Nations.

To learn more about Global Relay For Life or bring Relay to your organization, please visit *RelayForLife.org/global* or contact *globalrelay forlifemovement@cancer.org*.

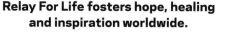

Relay For Life fosters hope, healing and inspiration worldwide.

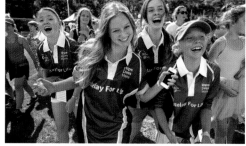
Relayers celebrate in Australia

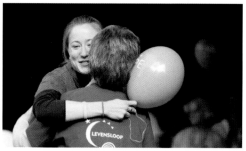
Fighting back in Belgium

Fostering hope

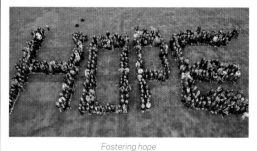
Remembering loved ones in Japan

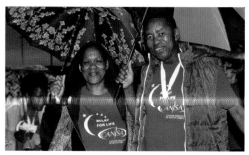
Survivors in Polokwane, South Africa

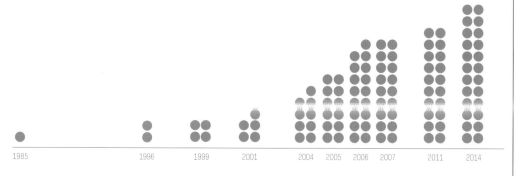

(1)

Participation in Global Relay For Life has grown steadily since 1996.

NUMBER OF COUNTRIES PARTICIPATING, BY YEAR

1985 1996 1999 2001 2004 2005 2006 2007 2011 2014

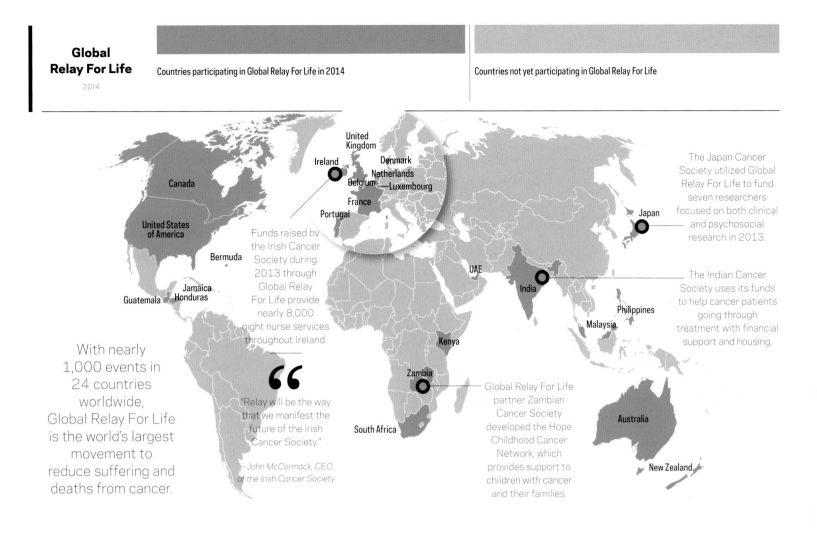

Global Relay For Life
2014

Countries participating in Global Relay For Life in 2014

Countries not yet participating in Global Relay For Life

United Kingdom
Ireland
Denmark
Netherlands
Belgium — Luxembourg
France
Portugal
Canada
United States of America
Bermuda
Jamaica
Honduras
Guatemala
UAE
India
Japan
Philippines
Malaysia
Kenya
Zambia
South Africa
Australia
New Zealand

The Japan Cancer Society utilized Global Relay For Life to fund seven researchers focused on both clinical and psychosocial research in 2013.

The Indian Cancer Society uses its funds to help cancer patients going through treatment with financial support and housing.

Funds raised by the Irish Cancer Society during 2013 through Global Relay For Life provide nearly 8,000 night nurse services throughout Ireland.

With nearly 1,000 events in 24 countries worldwide, Global Relay For Life is the world's largest movement to reduce suffering and deaths from cancer.

"Relay will be the way that we manifest the future of the Irish Cancer Society."

—*John McCormack, CEO of the Irish Cancer Society*

Global Relay For Life partner Zambian Cancer Society developed the Hope Childhood Cancer Network, which provides support to children with cancer and their families.

---

②

The effect of countries participating in Global Relay For Life is exponential.

2012 YEAR IN REVIEW

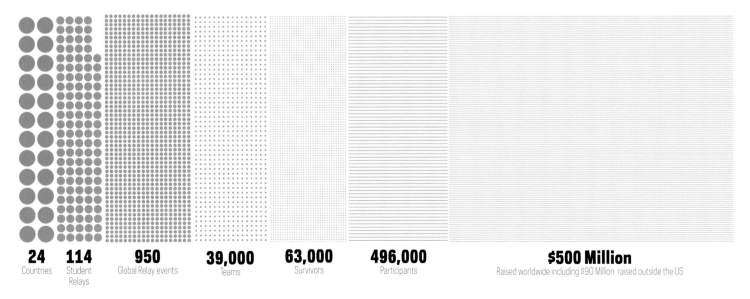

| **24** Countries | **114** Student Relays | **950** Global Relay events | **39,000** Teams | **63,000** Survivors | **496,000** Participants | **$500 Million** Raised worldwide including $90 Million raised outside the US |

POLICIES AND LEGISLATION

Globally and locally, policymakers use legislation and public policies to reduce leading risk factors, increase access to key technologies and services, and build enabling environments to improve health, well-being and development.

The World Health Organization Framework Convention on Tobacco Control (WHO FCTC) came into force in 2005, committing its parties to take action to reduce the single most preventable cause of cancer—tobacco use—and inspiring broader global action on non-communicable diseases (NCDs). ① In 2011, the United Nations General Assembly held a landmark high-level meeting to address chronic NCDs, including cancers, as a major development challenge. Leaders from over 120 nations committed to work to prevent, treat and manage these diseases, and in 2013 the World Health Assembly adopted the WHO Global Action Plan on NCDs, emphasizing whole-of-society approaches to reduce the major drivers of preventable cancer. ② The Plan also endorsed a global monitoring framework including nine voluntary global targets such as decreasing premature mortality from NCDs by 25% by 2025.

Meeting the global targets will require concerted national action. A recent WHO survey of 178 countries found that about two-thirds of countries currently have an operational policy, plan or strategy on cancer, either as a standalone plan (17%), integrated with other NCDs (17%), or both (33%). The WHO Global Action Plan on NCDs and the global monitoring framework will encourage countries to strengthen or develop national cancer plans with dedicated funding, strengthen cancer registries, reduce leading risk factors, and improve access to essential NCDs medicines and technologies, palliative care, cervical cancer screening, and vaccination.

Improved vaccine access is changing the global cancer prevention landscape. Over the last decade, major global public policy efforts have helped to bring about a twofold increase in the percentage of infants worldwide vaccinated against hepatitis B to prevent liver cancer later in life, with the most dramatic gains in the high-burden regions of Africa (from 23% to 72% coverage) and Southeast Asia (from 10% to 72% coverage). GAVI Alliance support to countries and negotiation of favorable pricing has enabled several low-income countries to vaccinate girls against the human papillomavirus (HPV) to protect them from developing cervical cancer. By negotiating for a common price that national ministries can afford, the Pan-American Health Organization's Revolving Fund also works to expand access to vaccines against cancer for low- and middle-income countries in the Americas.

Countries have also intensified cancer control efforts by passing strong tobacco control legislation and coordinating on global tobacco control concerns. The USA enacted new tobacco product regulatory authorities and implemented cutting-edge mobile communications and social media initiatives to help people quit smoking. In 2011, Australia limited tobacco marketing by legislatively mandating standardized plain packaging with large graphic warnings on all cigarettes. In 2012, Brazil became the most populous country to enact national indoor smoke-free legislation. The WHO FCTC Protocol to Eliminate Illicit Trade in Tobacco Products, adopted in 2012, requires parties to act domestically and cooperate internationally to control the supply chain.

"Addressing noncommunicable diseases (NCDs) is critical for global public health, but it will also be good for the economy; for the environment; for the global public good in the broadest sense. If we come together to tackle NCDs, we can do more than heal individuals— we can safeguard our very future."

— *UN Secretary General Ban Ki-moon*

Operational national cancer plans

2013

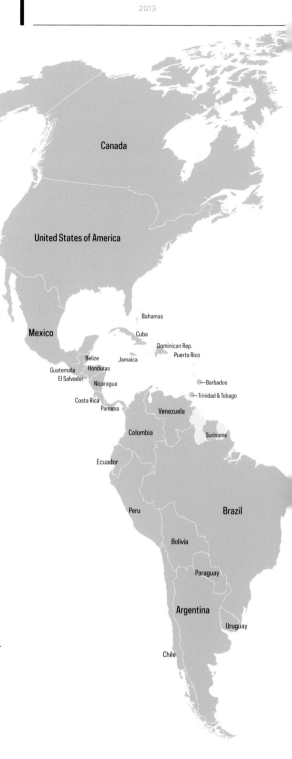

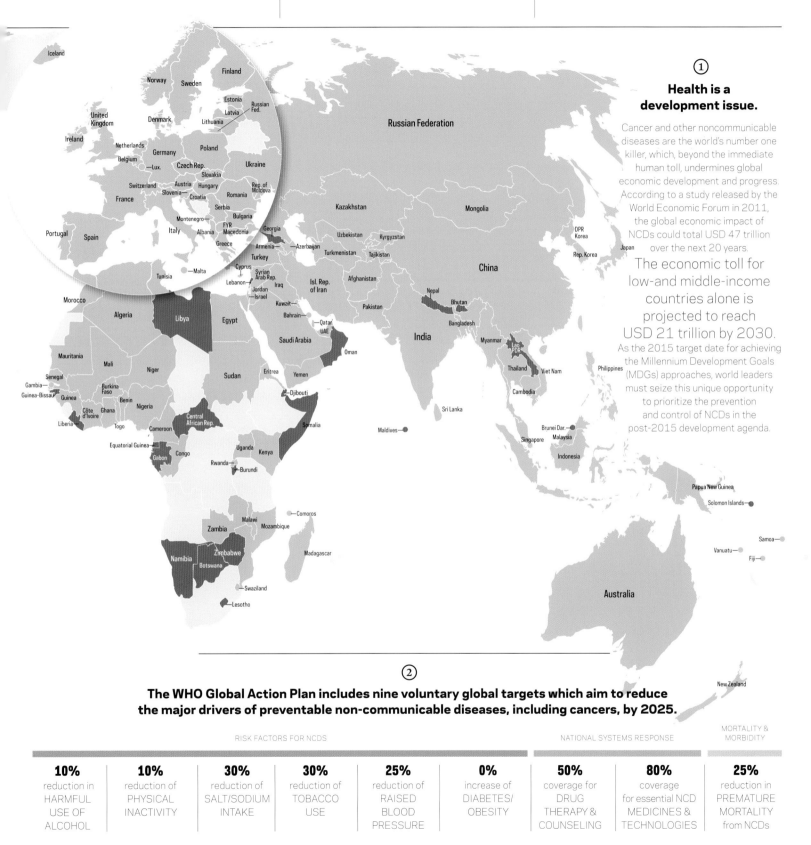

Countries with an operational national cancer plan

Countries without an operational national cancer plan

No Data

① **Health is a development issue.**

Cancer and other noncommunicable diseases are the world's number one killer, which, beyond the immediate human toll, undermines global economic development and progress. According to a study released by the World Economic Forum in 2011, the global economic impact of NCDs could total USD 47 trillion over the next 20 years.

The economic toll for low-and middle-income countries alone is projected to reach USD 21 trillion by 2030. As the 2015 target date for achieving the Millennium Development Goals (MDGs) approaches, world leaders must seize this unique opportunity to prioritize the prevention and control of NCDs in the post-2015 development agenda.

② **The WHO Global Action Plan includes nine voluntary global targets which aim to reduce the major drivers of preventable non-communicable diseases, including cancers, by 2025.**

RISK FACTORS FOR NCDS						NATIONAL SYSTEMS RESPONSE		MORTALITY & MORBIDITY
10% reduction in HARMFUL USE OF ALCOHOL	**10%** reduction of PHYSICAL INACTIVITY	**30%** reduction of SALT/SODIUM INTAKE	**30%** reduction of TOBACCO USE	**25%** reduction of RAISED BLOOD PRESSURE	**0%** increase of DIABETES/ OBESITY	**50%** coverage for DRUG THERAPY & COUNSELING	**80%** coverage for essential NCD MEDICINES & TECHNOLOGIES	**25%** reduction in PREMATURE MORTALITY from NCDs

BCE — 18TH CENTURY

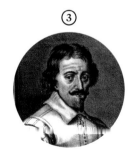

Hippocrates
FATHER OF MEDICINE

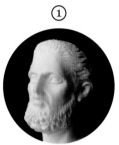

Christopher Columbus
BRINGS TOBACCO FROM AMERICAS TO EUROPE

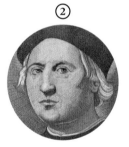

Zacharias Janssen
INVENTED THE COMPOUND MICROSCOPE

70 - 80 million years ago
Evidence of cancer cells in dinosaur fossils, found in 2003.

4.2 - 3.9 million years ago
The oldest known hominid malignant tumor was found in Homo erectus, or Australopithecus, by Louis Leakey in 1932.

3000 BCE
EGYPT

Evidence of cancerous cells found in mummies.

1900 - 1600 BCE
Cancer found in remains of Bronze Age human female skull.

1750 BCE
Babylonian code of Hammurabi set standard fee for surgical removal of tumors (ten shekels) and penalties for failure.

1600 BCE
EGYPT

The Egyptians blamed cancer on the gods. Ancient Egyptian scrolls describe eight cases of breast tumors treated by cauterization. Stomach cancer treated with boiled barley mixed with dates; cancer of the uterus by a concoction of fresh dates mixed with pig's brain introduced into the vagina.

1100 - 400 BCE
CHINA

China Physicians specializing in treating swellings and ulcerations were referred to in The Rites of the Zhou Dynasty.

500 BCE
INDIA

Indian epic tale, the Ramayana, described treatment with arsenic paste to thwart tumor growth.

400 BCE
PERU

Pre-Colombian Inca mummies found to contain lesions suggestive of malignant melanoma.

400 BCE
GREECE

① Greek physician Hippocrates (460-370 BCE), the "Father of Medicine," believed illness was caused by imbalance of four bodily humors: yellow bile, black bile, blood, and phlegm.

He was the first to recognize differences between benign and malignant tumors.

Circa 250 BCE
CHINA

The first clinical picture of breast cancer, including progression, metastasis, and death, and prognosis approximately ten years after diagnosis, was described in The Nei Ching, or The Yellow Emperor's Classic of Internal Medicine. It gave the first description of tumors and five forms of therapy: spiritual, pharmacological, diet, acupuncture, and treatment of respiratory diseases.

50 AD
ITALY

The Romans found some tumors could be removed by surgery and cauterized, but thought medicine did not work. They noted some tumors grew again.

100 AD
ITALY

Greek doctor Claudius Galen (129-216 AD) removed some tumors surgically, but he generally believed that cancer was best left untreated. Galen believed melancholia the chief factor in causing breast cancer, and recommended special diets, exorcism, and topical applications.

500 - 1500
EUROPE

Surgery and cautery were used on smaller tumors. Caustic pastes, usually containing arsenic, were used on more extensive cancers, as well as phlebotomy (blood-letting), diet, herbal medicines, powder of crab, and symbolic charms.

1400 - 1500s
ITALY

Leonardo da Vinci (1452-1519) dissected cadavers for artistic and scientific purposes, adding to the knowledge of the human body.

1492
EUROPE

② Christopher Columbus returned to Europe from the Americas with the first tobacco leaves and seeds ever seen on the continent. A crew member, Rodrigo de Jerez, was seen smoking and was imprisoned by the Inquisition, which believed he was possessed by the devil.

1500
EUROPE

Autopsies were conducted more often and understanding of internal cancers grew.

1595

NETHERLANDS

③ Zacharias Janssen invented the compound microscope.

17th century

NETHERLANDS

Dutch surgeon Adrian Helvetius performed both lumpectomy and mastectomy, claiming this cured breast cancer.

17th century

GERMANY

Cancer surgery techniques improved, but lack of anesthesia and antiseptic conditions made surgery a risky choice. German surgeon Wilhelm Fabricius Hildanus (1560-1634) removed enlarged lymph nodes in breast cancer operations, while Johann Scultetus (1595-1645) performed total mastectomies.

17th century

FRANCE

Physician Claude Gendron (1663-1750) concluded that cancer arises locally as a hard, growing mass, untreatable with drugs, and that it must be removed with all its "filaments."

17th century

NETHERLANDS

Professor Hermann Boerhaave (1668-1738) believed inflammation could result in cancer.

17th - 18th centuries

NETHERLANDS

Antony van Leeuwenhoek (1632-1723) refined the single lens microscope and was the first to see blood cells and bacteria, aiding the better understanding of cells, blood, and lymphatic system— major steps in improving the understanding of cancer.

FRANCE

Physician Le Dran (1685-1770) first recognized that breast cancer could spread to the regional auxiliary lymph nodes, carrying a poorer prognosis.

1713

ITALY

③ Dr. Bernardino Ramazzini (1633-1714), a founder of occupational/industrial medicine, reported the virtual absence of cervical cancer and relatively high incidence of breast cancer in nuns. This observation was an important step toward identifying hormonal factors such as pregnancy and infections related to sexual contact in cancer risk, and was the first indication that lifestyle might affect the development of cancer.

1733 - 1788

FRANCE

Physicians and scientists performed systematic experiments on cancer, leading to oncology as a medical specialty. Two French scientists— physician Jean Astruc and chemist Bernard Peyrilhe— were key to these new investigations.

1761

ITALY

Giovanni Morgagni performed the first autopsies to relate the patient's illness to the science of disease, laying the foundation for modern pathology.

1761

UNITED KINGDOM

⑤ Dr. John Hill published "Cautions Against the Immoderate Use of Snuff," the first report linking tobacco and cancer.

1775

UNITED KINGDOM

Dr. Percival Pott of Saint Bartholomew's Hospital in London described cancer in chimney sweeps caused by soot collecting under the scrotum, the first indication that exposure to chemicals in the environment could cause cancer. This research led to many additional studies that identified other occupational carcinogens and thence to public health measures to reduce cancer risk.

1779

FRANCE

⑥ First cancer hospital founded in Reims. It was forced to move from the city because people believed cancer was contagious.

18th century

UNITED KINGDOM

Scottish surgeon John Hunter (1728-93) stated that tumors originated in the lymph system and then seeded around the body. He suggested that some cancers might be cured by surgery, especially those that had not invaded nearby tissue.

④

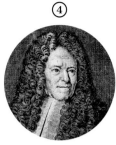

Dr. Bernardino Ramazzini
FOUNDER OF OCCUPATIONAL/INDUSTRIAL MEDICINE

⑤

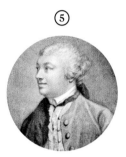

Dr. John Hill
PUBLISHED FIRST REPORT LINKING TOBACCO AND CANCER

⑥

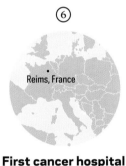

Reims, France

First cancer hospital
FOUNDED 1779

19TH CENTURY

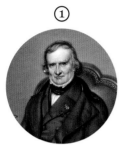

Joseph Recamier
COINED THE TERM "METASTASIS"

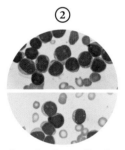

Leukemia described as a proliferation of blood cells
BY JOHN HUGHES BENNETT

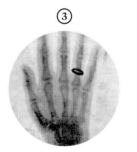

First x-ray
DISCOVERED BY WILHELM KONRAD ROENTGEN

19th century
UNITED KINGDOM

In the early 1800s, Scottish physician John Waldrop proposed that "glioma of the retina," which typically appeared within the eyes of newborns and young children and was usually lethal, might be cured via early removal of affected organs.

1829
FRANCE

① Gynecologist Joseph Recamier described the invasion of the bloodstream by cancer cells, coining the term metastasis, which came to mean the distant spread of cancer from its primary site to other places in the body.

1838
GERMANY

Pathologist Johannes Müller demonstrated that cancer is made up of cells and not lymph. His student, Rudolph Virchow (1821-1902), later proposed that chronic inflammation— the site of a wound that never heals— was the cause of cancer.

1842
ITALY

Domenico Antonio Rigoni-Stern undertook the first major statistical analysis of cancer incidence and mortality using 1760-1839 data from Verona. This showed that more women than men died from tumors, and that the most common female cancers were breast and uterine (each accounting for a third of total deaths). He found cancer death rates for both sexes were rising, and concluded that incidence of cancer increases with age, that cancer is found less in the country than in the city, and that unmarried people are more likely to contract the disease.

1845
UNITED KINGDOM

② John Hughes Bennett, the Edinburgh physician, was the first to describe leukemia as an excessive proliferation of blood cells.

1851-1971
UNITED KINGDOM

Decennial reports linked cancer death to occupation and social class.

1880

Earlier invention of general anesthesia (chloroform, ether, nitrous oxide) became more widespread, making cancer surgery more acceptable.

1881
USA

First practical cigarette-making machine patented by James Bonsack. It could produce 120,000 cigarettes a day, each machine doing the work of 48 people. Production costs plummeted, and— with the invention of the safety match a few decades later— cigarette smoking began its explosive growth.

1886
BRAZIL

Hereditary basis for cancer first suggested after Professor Hilario de Gouvea of the Medical School in Rio de Janeiro reported a family with increased susceptibility to retinoblastoma.

1890s
USA

Professor William Stewart Halsted at Johns Hopkins University developed the radical mastectomy for breast cancer, removing breast, underlying muscles, and lymph nodes under the arm.

1895
GERMANY

③ Physicist Wilhelm Konrad Roentgen (1845-1923) discovered x-rays, used in the diagnosis of cancer. Within a few years, this led to the use of radiation for cancer treatment.

1897
USA

Walter B. Cannon (1871-1945) was still a college student when he fed bismuth and barium mixtures to geese, outlining their gullets on an x-ray plate (the forerunner of the barium meal examination).

19th century

Invention and use of the modern microscope, which later helped identify cancer cells.

19th century
GERMANY

Rudolph Virchow (1821-1902), "the founder of cellular pathology," also determined that all cells, including cancer cells, are derived from other cells. He was the first to coin the term "leukemia" and believed that chronic inflammation was the cause of cancer.

19th century
GERMANY

Surgeon Karl Thiersch showed that cancers metastasize through the spread of malignant cells.

19th century
UNITED KINGDOM

Surgeon Stephen Paget (1855-1926) first deduced that cancer cells spread to all organs of the body by the bloodstream, but only grow in the organ ("soil") they find compatible. This laid the groundwork for the true understanding of metastasis.

1895
UNITED KINGDOM

Dr. Thomas Beatson discovered that the breasts of rabbits stopped producing milk after he removed the ovaries. This control of one organ over another led Beatson to test what would happen if the ovaries were removed in patients suffering from advanced breast cancer, and he found that oophorectomy often resulted in improvement. He thus discovered the stimulating effect of estrogen on breast tumors long before the hormone was discovered. This work provided a foundation for the modern use of hormones and analogs (e.g. tamoxifen, taxol) for treatment and prevention of breast cancer.

Before 1900

Lung cancer was extremely rare; now it is one of the most common cancers.

20TH CENTURY

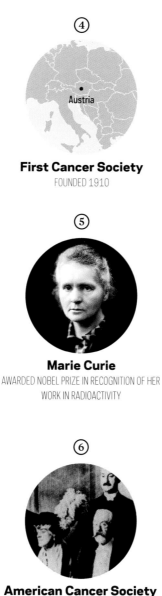

④

First Cancer Society
FOUNDED 1910

⑤

Marie Curie
AWARDED NOBEL PRIZE IN RECOGNITION OF HER WORK IN RADIOACTIVITY

⑥

American Cancer Society
FOUNDED 1913

By 1900

Hundreds of materials, both man-made and natural, were recognized as causes of cancer (carcinogens).

1902

X-ray exposure led to skin cancer on the hand of a lab technician. Within a decade, many more physicians and scientists, unaware of the dangers of radiation, developed a variety of cancers.

1905
UNITED KINGDOM

Physicians at the Royal Ophthalmology Hospital reported the first case of "hereditary" retinal glioma, which presented in the child of a parent cured of the disease.

1907
USA

Epidemiological study found that meat-eating Germans, Irish, and Scandinavians living in Chicago had higher rates of cancer than did Italians and Chinese, who ate considerably less meat.

1910
AUSTRIA

④ First national cancer society founded: Austrian Cancer Society.

1911
FRANCE

⑤ Marie Curie was awarded a second Nobel Prize, this time in chemistry, in recognition of her work in radioactivity.

1900 - 1950

Radiotherapy— the use of radiation to kill cancer cells or stop them dividing— was developed as a treatment.

1911
USA

Peyotn Rous (1879-1970) proved that viruses caused cancer in chickens, for which he was eventually awarded the Nobel Prize in 1966.

1913
USA

⑥ The American Cancer Society was founded as the American Society for the Control of Cancer (ASCC) by 15 physicians and business leaders in New York City. In 1945, the ASCC was renamed the American Cancer Society. It remains the world's largest voluntary health organization.

1915
JAPAN

Cancer was induced in laboratory animals for the first time by a chemical, coal tar, applied to rabbits' skin at Tokyo University. Soon many other substances were observed to be carcinogens, including benzene, hydrocarbons, aniline, asbestos, and tobacco.

1926
UNITED KINGDOM

(1) Physician and epidemiologist Janet Lane-Claypon (1877-1967) published results from a study that demonstrated some of the major contemporary risk factors for breast cancer among women, including not breastfeeding, being childless, and older age at first pregnancy.

1928
GREECE

(2) George Papanicolaou (1883-1962) identified malignant cells among the normal cast-off vaginal cells of women with cancer of the cervix, which led to the Pap smear test.

1930
GERMANY

Researchers in Cologne drew the first statistical connection between smoking and cancer.

1930s
PUERTO RICO

Dr. Cornelius Rhoads, a pathologist, allegedly injected his Puerto Rican subjects with cancer cells—13 people died.

1933

The Union for International Cancer Control (UICC) founded.

1933
SPAIN

First World Cancer Congress held in Madrid.

1930s - 1950s

Classification of breast cancer introduced, enabling the planning of more rational treatment tailored to the individual.

1934
UNITED KINGDOM

Drs. W. Burton Wood and S. R. Gloyne reported the first two cases of lung cancer linked to asbestos.

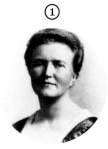

Janet Lane-Claypon
PUBLISHED RISK FACTORS IN BREAST CANCER

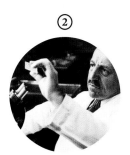

George Papanicolaou
CONDUCTS FIRST PAP SMEAR

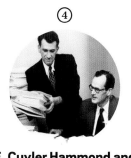

Gertrude Elion
CREATED NEW LEUKEMIA TREATMENT

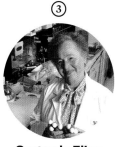

E. Cuyler Hammond and Daniel Horn
LAUNCHED THE HAMMOND-HORN STUDY

1937
USA

National Cancer Institute inaugurated.

1939
USA

Drs. Alton Ochsner and Michael DeBakey first reported the association of smoking and lung cancer.

1939 - 1945

During the Second World War, the US Army discovered that nitrogen mustard was effective in treating cancer of the lymph nodes (lymphoma). This was the birth of chemotherapy— the use of drugs to treat cancer.

1943 - 1945
DENMARK, UNITED KINGDOM

First national cancer registries established.

1947
CANADA

Dr. Norman Delarue compared 50 patients with lung cancer with 50 patients hospitalized with other diseases. He discovered that over 90% of the first group— but only half of the second— were smokers, and confidently predicted that by 1950 no one would be smoking.

1947
USA

Sidney Farber (1903-73), one of the founders of the specialty of pediatric pathology, used a derivative of folic acid, methotrexate, to inhibit acute leukemia in children.

1940s - 1950s
USA

Dr. Charles B. Huggins' (1901-97) research on prostate cancer changed the way scientists regard the behavior of all cancer cells, and for the first time brought hope to the prospect of treating advanced cancers. He showed that cancer cells were not autonomous and self-perpetuating but were dependent on chemical signals such as hormones to grow and survive, and that depriving cancer cells of these signals could restore the health of patients with widespread metastases. He was awarded the Nobel Prize in 1966 (shared with Peyton Rous).

1950
USA

③ Gertrude Elion (1918-99) created a purine chemical, which she developed into 6-mercaptopurine, or 6-MP. It was rapidly approved for use in childhood leukemia. She received the Nobel Prize in 1988.

1950
USA

The link between smoking and lung cancer was confirmed. A landmark article from *The Journal of the American Medical Association* appeared on May 27th, 1950: "Tobacco smoking as a possible etiologic factor in bronchogenic carcinoma" by E.L. Wynder and Evarts Graham. The same issue featured a full-page ad for Chesterfields with the actress Gene Tierney and golfer Ben Hogan; the journal accepted tobacco ads until 1953.

1951
UNITED KINGDOM

Dr. Richard Doll and Prof. Austin Bradford Hill conducted the first large-scale study of the link between smoking and lung cancer.

1952
USA

④ Epidemiologists at the American Cancer Society launched the Hammond-Horn Study, a long-term follow-up study of 188,000 men designed to examine the association of cigarette smoking with death from cancer and other diseases.

1953
UNITED KINGDOM

James Watson and Francis Crick described the double helical structure of DNA, marking the beginning of the modern era of genetics.

1954
USA

⑤ First tobacco litigation against the cigarette companies, brought by a widow on behalf of her smoker husband, who died from cancer. The cigarette companies won.

1956
USA

⑥ Dr. Min Chiu Li (1919-1980) first demonstrated clinically that chemotherapy could result in the cure of a widely metastatic malignant disease.

1960
JAPAN

Group cancer screening for stomach cancer began with a mobile clinic in Tohoku region.

⑤

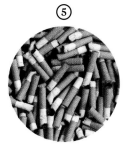

First tobacco litigation against the cigarette companies

⑥

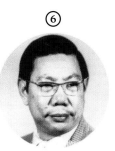

Dr. Min Chiu Li
FIRST DEMONSTRATED CHEMOTHERAPY AS A CURE

⑦

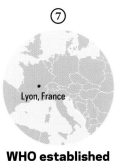

Lyon, France

WHO established International Agency for Research on Cancer
FOUNDED IN 1965

⑧

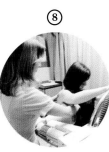

Mammography screening trials

1960
USA

Dr. Min Chiu Li published another important and original finding: the use of multiple-agent combination chemotherapy for the treatment of metastatic cancers of the testis. Twenty years later, it was demonstrated that combination chemotherapy, combined with techniques for local control, had virtually eliminated deaths from testicular malignancy.

1963
JAPAN

Cancer research programs were established by the Ministry of Health and Welfare and the Ministry of Education, Science, and Culture.

1964
USA

Physician Irving J. Selikoff (1915-92) published the results from a study linking asbestos exposure to the development of mesothelioma.

1964
USA

First US Surgeon General's report on smoking and health.

1965
FRANCE

⑦ WHO established the International Agency for Research on Cancer (IARC), based in Lyon, France.

1966

International Association of Cancer Registries (IACR) founded.

1960s - 1970s

⑧ Trials in several countries demonstrated the effectiveness of mammography screening for breast cancer.

1970s
USA, ITALY

Bernard Fisher in the USA and Umberto Veronesi in Italy both launched long-term studies as to whether lumpectomy followed by radiation therapy was an alternative to radical mastectomy in early breast cancer. These studies concluded that total mastectomy offered no advantage over either lumpectomy or lumpectomy plus radiation therapy.

1971

USA

The National Cancer Act in President Nixon's "War on Cancer" mandated financial support for cancer research, outlined intervention strategies, and, in 1973, established the Surveillance, Epidemiology, and End Results (SEER) program, a network of population-based cancer registries.

1973

USA

Bone marrow transplantation first performed successfully on a dog in Seattle by Dr. E. Donnall Thomas (1920–2012). This led to human bone marrow transplantation, resulting in cures for leukemias and lymphomas. In 1990, Dr. Thomas won a Nobel Prize for his work.

1970s

Childhood leukemia became one of the first cancers that could be cured by a combination of drugs.

1970s

USA

Discovery of the first cancer gene (the oncogene, which in certain circumstances can transform a cell into a tumor cell).

1970s onwards

WHO, UICC, and others promoted national cancer planning for nations to prioritize and focus their cancer control activities.

1981

JAPAN

Professor Takeshi Hirayama (1923–95) published the first report linking passive smoking and lung cancer in the non-smoking wives of men who smoked.

1981

ITALY

Dr. G. Bonnadona in Milan performed the first study of adjuvant chemotherapy for breast cancer using cyclophosphamide, methotrexate, and 5-fluorouracil, resulting in reduction of cancer relapse. Adjuvant chemotherapy is now standard treatment for lung, breast, colon, stomach, and ovary cancers.

1980s

USA

Kaposi's sarcoma and T-cell lymphoma linked to AIDS.

1982

USA

Nobel Laureate Baruch S. Blumberg was instrumental in developing a reliable and safe vaccine against hepatitis B (which causes primary liver cancer).

1980s

AUSTRALIA

Barry Marshall and J. Robin Warren identified bacterium *H. pylori*, noting it caused duodenal and gastric ulcers and increased the risk of gastric cancer.

1980s

USA

Vincent DeVita developed a four-drug combination to significantly raise the cure rate of Hodgkin disease to 80%.

Mid - 1980s

Human Genome Project was initiated to pinpoint location and function of estimated 50,000–100,000 genes that make up the inherited set of "instructions" for functions and behavior of human beings.

1980s

WHO Program on Cancer Control established.

1988

First WHO World No Tobacco Day, subsequently an annual event.

1989

European Network of Cancer Registries (ENCR) established.

1989

USA

National Institutes of Health researchers performed the first approved gene therapy, inserting foreign genes to track tumor-killing cells in cancer patients. This project proved the safety of gene therapy.

1991

Evidence linking specific environmental carcinogens to telltale DNA damage emerged, e.g. sub radiation was found to produce change in tumor suppressor genes in skin cells, aflatoxin (a fungus poison) or hepatitis B virus to cause a mutation in the liver, and chemicals in cigarette smoke to switch on a gene that makes lung cells vulnerable to the chemicals' cancer-causing properties.

1994

USA, CANADA, UNITED KINGDOM, FRANCE, JAPAN

Scientists collaborated and discovered BRCA1, the first known breast and ovarian cancer predisposing gene.

1994

USA

National Program of Cancer Registries (NPCR) established.

1995

Gene therapy, immune system modulation, and genetically engineered antibodies used to treat cancer.

1999

NETHERLANDS, USA

Jan Walboomers of the Free University of Amsterdam and Michele Manos of Johns Hopkins University provided evidence that the human papillomavirus (HPV) is present in 99.7% of all cases of cervical cancer.

1999

The Bill & Melinda Gates Foundation awarded a five-year, $50 million grant to the Alliance for Cervical Cancer Prevention (ACCP), a group of five international organizations with a shared goal of working to prevent cervical cancer in developing countries.

21ST CENTURY

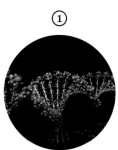

Human genome is mapped

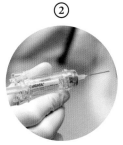

First HPV vaccine

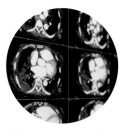

CT scan screening for lung cancer

2000

53rd World Health Assembly presided over by Dr. Libertina Amathila (Namibia) endorsed "Global strategy for non-communicable disease (NCD) prevention and control," which outlined major objectives for monitoring, preventing, and managing NCDs, with special emphasis on major NCDs with common risk factors and determinants— cardiovascular disease, cancer, diabetes, and chronic respiratory disease.

2000

① The entire human genome is mapped.

2000

Charter of Paris against Cancer is signed.

2001

LUXEMBOURG

International Childhood Cancer Day was launched, its aim to raise awareness of the 250,000 children worldwide who get cancer every year. Some 80% of these children have little or no access to treatment. The first annual event in 2002 was supported in 30 countries around the world and raised over US$100,000 for parent organizations to help children in their own countries.

2004

SWITZERLAND

WHO cancer prevention and control resolution approved by World Health Assembly.

2005

WHO Framework Convention on Tobacco Control came into force, using international law to further public health and prevent cancer.

2006

USA

② The US Federal Drug Administration approved the first HPV vaccine to prevent infections that cause cervical cancer.

2011

③ Lung cancer deaths reduced by low-dose computed tomography (CT) scanning of people at high risk.

2011

UN High Level Meeting on Non-communicable Diseases in New York, USA.

RISK FACTORS FOR CANCER

Countries	Population IN THOUSANDS	Youth smoking prevalence (%), AGES 10-14 YEARS, 2013		Adult smoking prevalence (%), AGES 15+ YEARS, 2013	
		Male	Female	Male	Female
Afghanistan	28,398	1.0%	0.4%	22.9%	2.8%
Albania	3,150	1.1%	0.2%	38.4%	4.0%
Algeria	37,063	6.6%	0.4%	21.7%	0.9%
Angola	19,549	0.1%	0.3%	16.7%	1.6%
Argentina	40,374	2.1%	2.7%	23.8%	15.7%
Armenia	2,963	1.3%	0.1%	51.7%	1.8%
Australia	22,404	2.3%	3.8%	18.5%	15.6%
Austria	8,402	3.7%	4.0%	36.5%	28.5%
Azerbaijan	9,095	0.6%	0.1%	44.9%	0.9%
Bahamas	360	0.7%	0.3%	15.8%	4.5%
Bahrain	1,252	2.2%	0.8%	23.8%	6.1%
Bangladesh	151,125	1.2%	0.1%	44.4%	1.8%
Barbados	280	4.6%	2.2%	10.7%	2.1%
Belarus	9,491	6.6%	3.8%	46.0%	12.1%
Belgium	10,941	5.8%	8.3%	30.8%	26.2%
Belize	309	0.5%	0.2%	17.4%	1.8%
Benin	9,510	3.6%	1.4%	13.7%	1.9%
Bhutan	717	1.7%	0.7%	16.7%	3.5%
Bolivia (Plurinational State of)	10,157	4.7%	2.7%	38.6%	11.2%
Bosnia and Herzegovina	3,846	2.5%	0.8%	39.8%	24.3%
Botswana	1,969	2.7%	2.1%	21.5%	6.1%
Brazil	195,210	1.4%	0.9%	16.6%	11.1%
Brunei Darussalam	401	1.4%	1.3%	14.0%	8.4%
Bulgaria	7,389	4.3%	7.0%	40.8%	31.5%
Burkina Faso	15,540	1.1%	0.1%	19.8%	3.8%
Burundi	9,233	0.4%	0.2%	24.6%	9.8%
Cambodia	14,365	0.8%	0.6%	42.0%	4.0%
Cameroon	20,624	0.5%	0.0%	15.4%	0.6%
Canada	34,126	2.6%	2.9%	16.7%	12.9%
Cape Verde	488	0.3%	0.2%	11.6%	3.2%
Central African Republic	4,350	0.1%	0.3%	15.9%	1.5%
Chad	11,721	0.7%	0.4%	14.1%	2.3%
Chile	17,151	4.8%	5.4%	32.1%	26.3%
China	1,359,821	2.3%	0.2%	45.3%	2.1%
Colombia	46,445	3.0%	1.7%	17.3%	5.6%
Comoros	683	0.4%	0.5%	18.1%	2.5%
Congo	4,112	0.1%	0.3%	16.2%	1.4%
Congo (Democratic Republic of)	62,191	0.1%	0.3%	15.3%	1.4%
Costa Rica	4,670	3.2%	2.6%	16.0%	7.5%
Côte d'Ivoire	18,977	0.3%	0.2%	18.7%	1.8%
Croatia	4,338	6.2%	8.2%	38.0%	24.5%
Cuba	11,282	0.7%	0.8%	19.9%	11.8%
Cyprus	1,104	5.9%	2.9%	48.1%	18.4%
Czech Republic	10,554	2.0%	3.5%	28.7%	20.3%
Denmark	5,551	2.8%	3.4%	19.9%	17.8%
Djibouti	834	2.1%	0.5%	38.9%	7.4%

Prevalence (%) of overweight and obesity (BMI>25), 2008		Percentage of one-year-olds* GIVEN THE 3-SERIES HEPATITIS B VACCINATION, 2012	The risk of getting cancer: PROBABILITY OF DEVELOPING A CANCER BEFORE AGE 75, 2012	Countries
Male	**Female**			
10.0%	13.6%	71%	12.2%	Afghanistan
60.5%	48.2%	99%	18.4%	Albania
41.8%	54.5%	95%	12.8%	Algeria
20.4%	30.7%	91%	10.8%	Angola
66.8%	61.1%	91%	21.8%	Argentina
49.2%	59.3%	95%	25.8%	Armenia
66.5%	56.2%	92%	31.0%	Australia
56.9%	42.1%	83%	25.5%	Austria
52.0%	61.9%	46%	15.2%	Azerbaijan
66.0%	72.1%	96%	21.0%	Bahamas
70.2%	70.5%	99%	12.0%	Bahrain
7.6%	7.8%	96%	11.2%	Bangladesh
60.8%	75.1%	88%	25.3%	Barbados
56.7%	55.6%	97%	22.9%	Belarus
59.8%	43.1%	98%	31.4%	Belgium
65.4%	76.6%	98%	16.7%	Belize
20.4%	31.7%	85%	9.6%	Benin
24.5%	24.4%	97%	8.6%	Bhutan
40.4%	58.9%	80%	14.7%	Bolivia (Plurinational State of)
61.9%	53.1%	92%	17.3%	Bosnia and Herzegovina
18.3%	52.3%	96%	10.6%	Botswana
53.5%	52.0%	97%	20.8%	Brazil
35.8%	24.6%	99%	17.7%	Brunei Darussalam
61.2%	47.1%	95%	23.8%	Bulgaria
11.9%	14.2%	90%	9.1%	Burkina Faso
16.0%	14.7%	96%	14.3%	Burundi
11.4%	13.8%	95%	14.7%	Cambodia
32.6%	42.3%	85%	9.6%	Cameroon
65.7%	55.2%	70%	29.1%	Canada
30.8%	42.6%	90%	7.5%	Cape Verde
12.4%	20.9%	47%	9.9%	Central African Republic
14.6%	16.9%	45%	9.1%	Chad
64.2%	65.7%	90%	18.0%	Chile
25.1%	24.9%	99%	16.8%	China
44.9%	53.8%	92%	16.6%	Colombia
19.4%	21.1%	86%	10.7%	Comoros
16.9%	27.0%	85%	10.2%	Congo
6.1%	14.5%	72%	12.0%	Congo (Democratic Republic of)
60.3%	58.8%	91%	18.2%	Costa Rica
21.8%	32.3%	94%	9.0%	Côte d'Ivoire
61.6%	44.6%	98%	26.5%	Croatia
47.5%	57.9%	96%	22.5%	Cuba
64.6%	47.6%	96%	20.6%	Cyprus
69.9%	53.1%	99%	29.3%	Czech Republic
54.6%	42.1%	0%	32.9%	Denmark
30.2%	37.4%	81%	9.8%	Djibouti

*Countries with 0% coverage may represent countries where hepatitis B is not endemic (e.g. Scandinavian countries) and national hepatitis B vaccination programs have not been introduced.

103

RISK FACTORS FOR CANCER

Countries	Population IN THOUSANDS	Youth smoking prevalence (%), AGES 10-14 YEARS, 2013		Adult smoking prevalence (%), AGES 15+ YEARS, 2013	
		Male	Female	Male	Female
Dominican Republic	10,017	0.2%	0.3%	14.5%	9.6%
Ecuador	15,001	0.5%	0.3%	10.4%	3.0%
Egypt	78,076	0.9%	0.2%	36.1%	1.2%
El Salvador	6,218	0.7%	0.1%	18.2%	2.6%
Equatorial Guinea	696	0.1%	0.1%	16.4%	1.5%
Eritrea	5,741	0.3%	0.2%	11.3%	0.6%
Estonia	1,299	5.6%	3.2%	38.8%	18.7%
Ethiopia	87,095	0.2%	0.1%	7.7%	1.0%
Fiji	861	7.1%	1.9%	23.4%	4.6%
Finland	5,368	6.4%	6.5%	20.6%	15.5%
France	63,231	2.9%	4.1%	34.4%	27.9%
French Guiana	231	-	-	-	-
French Polynesia	268	-	-	-	-
Gabon	1,556	1.1%	0.9%	19.1%	2.9%
Gambia	1,681	0.9%	0.5%	24.9%	0.8%
Georgia	4,389	1.2%	0.7%	45.3%	4.5%
Germany	83,017	5.7%	5.5%	28.0%	22.2%
Ghana	24,263	0.7%	0.7%	8.3%	1.3%
Greece	11,110	1.9%	1.4%	41.0%	34.7%
Greenland	57	-	-	-	-
Guadeloupe	459	-	-	-	-
Guam	159	-	-	-	-
Guatemala	14,342	0.6%	0.5%	11.7%	2.1%
Guinea	10,876	0.9%	0.4%	12.0%	1.6%
Guinea-Bissau	1,587	0.7%	0.4%	12.5%	2.0%
Guyana	786	1.0%	0.9%	27.9%	3.5%
Haiti	9,896	1.1%	0.6%	13.1%	3.4%
Honduras	7,621	1.3%	0.6%	20.6%	1.9%
Hungary	10,015	14.6%	10.4%	31.3%	25.4%
Iceland	318	2.3%	2.6%	15.9%	13.1%
India	1,205,625	0.2%	0.1%	23.2%	3.2%
Indonesia	240,676	1.9%	0.1%	57.1%	3.6%
Iran (Islamic Republic of)	74,462	0.3%	0.2%	23.3%	1.7%
Iraq	30,962	3.3%	0.9%	33.1%	2.9%
Ireland	4,468	3.2%	3.0%	25.1%	24.3%
Israel	7,420	3.5%	1.2%	26.1%	14.1%
Italy	60,509	3.5%	4.0%	27.3%	22.0%
Jamaica	2,741	0.9%	0.8%	26.9%	3.9%
Japan	127,353	2.0%	0.8%	35.5%	11.2%
Jordan	6,455	1.6%	0.5%	43.3%	8.5%
Kazakhstan	15,921	1.7%	0.6%	43.1%	6.4%
Kenya	40,909	0.5%	0.8%	20.2%	1.4%
Korea (Democratic People's Republic of)	24,501	3.4%	1.1%	45.8%	2.6%
Korea (Republic of)	48,454	2.5%	1.2%	42.2%	5.9%
Kuwait	2,992	3.7%	0.6%	31.3%	3.4%
Kyrgyzstan	5,334	0.6%	0.2%	35.8%	3.3%

Prevalence (%) of overweight and obesity (BMI>25), 2008		Percentage of one-year-olds* GIVEN THE 3-SERIES HEPATITIS B VACCINATION, 2012	The risk of getting cancer: PROBABILITY OF DEVELOPING A CANCER BEFORE AGE 75, 2012	Countries
Male	**Female**			
49.6%	61.1%	74%	15.7%	Dominican Republic
51.8%	60.2%	98%	16.5%	Ecuador
62.4%	76.9%	93%	15.4%	Egypt
59.1%	65.6%	92%	15.2%	El Salvador
33.0%	38.9%	0%	8.9%	Equatorial Guinea
9.6%	11.4%	99%	10.5%	Eritrea
57.8%	45.0%	94%	25.2%	Estonia
7.1%	9.0%	61%	11.1%	Ethiopia
60.1%	72.9%	99%	13.4%	Fiji
59.6%	46.2%	0%	25.9%	Finland
52.0%	40.0%	74%	32.0%	France
-	-	-	16.3%	French Guiana
-	-	-	26.5%	French Polynesia
36.5%	51.6%	82%	9.7%	Gabon
14.9%	40.9%	98%	4.6%	Gambia
50.7%	54.8%	92%	18.7%	Georgia
62.8%	46.6%	86%	28.3%	Germany
24.2%	36.7%	92%	9.3%	Ghana
56.6%	41.3%	98%	16.0%	Greece
-	-	-	-	Greenland
-	-	-	21.1%	Guadeloupe
-	-	-	17.6%	Guam
48.6%	58.6%	96%	13.3%	Guatemala
22.2%	20.8%	59%	9.7%	Guinea
15.3%	26.3%	76%	8.2%	Guinea-Bissau
34.6%	56.6%	97%	17.2%	Guyana
35.0%	29.4%	0%	10.7%	Haiti
46.7%	57.8%	88%	13.3%	Honduras
65.8%	49.4%	0%	28.3%	Hungary
63.6%	49.1%	0%	28.7%	Iceland
10.0%	12.5%	70%	10.1%	India
16.1%	25.3%	64%	14.0%	Indonesia
48.8%	61.0%	98%	13.1%	Iran (Islamic Republic of)
62.2%	68.2%	77%	14.4%	Iraq
67.1%	54.8%	95%	30.2%	Ireland
62.5%	57.8%	97%	28.1%	Israel
58.3%	40.1%	97%	27.4%	Italy
40.7%	70.6%	99%	21.1%	Jamaica
28.9%	15.9%	0%	21.8%	Japan
66.5%	71.2%	98%	16.1%	Jordan
57.0%	55.9%	95%	23.9%	Kazakhstan
15.2%	25.5%	83%	19.0%	Kenya
19.6%	15.3%	96%	19.2%	Korea (Democratic People's Republic of)
33.4%	27.4%	99%	29.3%	Korea (Republic of)
78.1%	81.3%	98%	11.1%	Kuwait
43.4%	48.9%	96%	14.9%	Kyrgyzstan

*Countries with 0% coverage may represent countries where hepatitis B is not endemic (e.g. Scandinavian countries) and national hepatitis B vaccination programs have not been introduced.

105

RISK FACTORS FOR CANCER

Countries	Population IN THOUSANDS	Youth smoking prevalence (%), AGES 10-14 YEARS, 2013		Adult smoking prevalence (%), AGES 15+ YEARS, 2013	
		Male	Female	Male	Female
Lao People's Democratic Republic	6,396	0.7%	0.6%	51.3%	11.4%
Latvia	2,091	7.0%	5.2%	44.7%	19.3%
Lebanon	4,341	1.4%	0.6%	34.0%	21.2%
Lesotho	2,009	2.8%	1.2%	35.6%	1.0%
Liberia	3,958	0.2%	0.0%	13.2%	1.3%
Libya	6,041	1.1%	1.0%	29.5%	0.9%
Lithuania	3,068	6.5%	2.9%	40.6%	16.1%
Luxembourg	508	3.3%	3.3%	30.2%	22.9%
Macedonia (The former Yugoslav Republic of)	2,102	1.3%	1.2%	46.6%	26.8%
Madagascar	21,080	1.6%	0.4%	26.6%	1.6%
Malawi	15,014	0.6%	0.1%	21.9%	2.7%
Malaysia	28,276	9.6%	1.0%	37.9%	1.4%
Maldives	326	0.9%	2.2%	34.5%	7.7%
Mali	13,986	0.9%	0.3%	18.7%	3.9%
Malta	425	3.3%	4.3%	28.0%	18.9%
Martinique	401	-	-	-	-
Mauritania	3,609	3.2%	2.2%	21.7%	3.8%
Mauritius	1,231	11.5%	3.7%	34.0%	2.8%
Mexico	117,886	2.2%	0.9%	16.0%	5.2%
Moldova (Republic of)	3,573	5.0%	1.2%	39.4%	5.1%
Mongolia	2,713	5.7%	1.2%	45.0%	6.3%
Montenegro	620	0.6%	0.7%	34.6%	20.2%
Morocco	31,642	0.5%	0.2%	26.7%	0.8%
Mozambique	23,967	0.7%	0.1%	22.3%	4.2%
Myanmar	51,931	0.9%	0.2%	30.6%	6.5%
Namibia	2,179	2.2%	2.6%	24.5%	10.0%
Nepal	26,846	0.5%	0.3%	37.6%	16.7%
Netherlands	16,615	2.4%	3.2%	22.6%	20.5%
New Caledonia	246	-	-	-	-
New Zealand	4,368	5.0%	5.5%	18.6%	17.8%
Nicaragua	5,822	1.1%	0.5%	17.2%	5.7%
Niger	15,894	0.5%	0.3%	8.9%	1.6%
Nigeria	159,708	0.3%	0.1%	7.4%	1.4%
Norway	4,891	2.6%	3.3%	17.4%	16.1%
Oman	2,803	0.5%	0.7%	13.0%	0.9%
Pakistan	173,149	6.9%	1.2%	27.9%	5.4%
Panama	3,678	0.2%	0.2%	13.8%	3.3%
Papua New Guinea	6,859	7.1%	1.4%	51.2%	21.5%
Paraguay	6,460	0.5%	0.1%	19.3%	5.4%
Peru	29,263	0.4%	0.9%	17.9%	4.5%
Philippines	93,444	0.8%	0.4%	40.0%	8.2%
Poland	38,199	4.1%	3.8%	31.8%	24.0%
Portugal	10,590	2.2%	1.7%	31.9%	15.7%
Puerto Rico	3,710	-	-	-	-
Qatar	1,750	1.2%	0.3%	19.4%	1.4%
Reunion	845	-	-	-	-

Prevalence (%) of overweight and obesity (BMI>25), 2008		Percentage of one-year-olds* GIVEN THE 3-SERIES HEPATITIS B VACCINATION, 2012	The risk of getting cancer: PROBABILITY OF DEVELOPING A CANCER BEFORE AGE 75, 2012	Countries
Male	Female			
11.6%	17.8%	79%	15.1%	Lao People's Democratic Republic
59.4%	47.8%	91%	25.6%	Latvia
67.0%	58.7%	84%	19.4%	Lebanon
17.3%	58.1%	83%	10.0%	Lesotho
17.7%	27.5%	77%	9.4%	Liberia
60.4%	71.0%	98%	13.2%	Libya
62.8%	51.0%	93%	25.7%	Lithuania
64.0%	49.2%	95%	27.9%	Luxembourg
59.6%	46.0%	96%	24.7%	Macedonia (The former Yugoslav Republic of)
12.6%	8.8%	86%	14.6%	Madagascar
16.7%	24.3%	96%	14.6%	Malawi
42.4%	47.0%	98%	15.0%	Malaysia
29.4%	52.5%	99%	9.8%	Maldives
15.3%	25.7%	74%	11.6%	Mali
66.8%	56.0%	93%	23.7%	Malta
-	-	-	25.8%	Martinique
22.8%	53.9%	80%	8.5%	Mauritania
46.7%	51.7%	98%	18.0%	Mauritius
67.8%	70.3%	99%	13.4%	Mexico
38.7%	57.7%	94%	21.1%	Moldova (Republic of)
44.4%	49.6%	99%	21.7%	Mongolia
61.3%	48.4%	90%	24.3%	Montenegro
43.1%	53.6%	99%	12.6%	Morocco
16.5%	28.0%	76%	13.5%	Mozambique
13.8%	23.6%	38%	14.7%	Myanmar
23.3%	44.7%	84%	8.8%	Namibia
9.8%	8.9%	90%	9.2%	Nepal
52.4%	43.2%	0%	30.2%	Netherlands
-	-	-	29.5%	New Caledonia
67.8%	60.6%	93%	28.8%	New Zealand
53.3%	63.2%	98%	11.9%	Nicaragua
11.0%	16.6%	74%	6.7%	Niger
26.2%	31.2%	41%	10.4%	Nigeria
62.3%	47.6%	0%	31.5%	Norway
57.8%	57.2%	97%	8.9%	Oman
20.0%	28.8%	81%	11.8%	Pakistan
58.2%	64.1%	85%	14.9%	Panama
45.4%	50.3%	63%	17.0%	Papua New Guinea
50.9%	50.2%	87%	14.8%	Paraguay
43.3%	52.2%	95%	15.7%	Peru
24.5%	29.1%	70%	14.8%	Philippines
61.6%	49.6%	98%	23.8%	Poland
59.7%	50.8%	98%	24.4%	Portugal
-	-	-	21.6%	Puerto Rico
72.5%	71.3%	92%	12.5%	Qatar
-	-	-	20.1%	Reunion

*Countries with 0% coverage may represent countries where hepatitis B is not endemic (e.g. Scandinavian countries) and national hepatitis B vaccination programs have not been introduced.

RISK FACTORS FOR CANCER

Countries	Population IN THOUSANDS	Youth smoking prevalence (%), AGES 10-14 YEARS, 2013		Adult smoking prevalence (%), AGES 15+ YEARS, 2013	
		Male	Female	Male	Female
Romania	21,861	2.8%	2.1%	36.6%	18.5%
Russian Federation	143,618	6.1%	4.0%	51.0%	17.0%
Rwanda	10,837	0.7%	0.3%	16.3%	2.7%
Samoa	186	2.1%	1.0%	33.6%	13.3%
Saudi Arabia	27,258	1.6%	0.3%	22.2%	2.2%
Senegal	12,951	0.7%	0.2%	14.5%	1.2%
Serbia	9,647	1.3%	1.0%	31.8%	22.8%
Sierra Leone	5,752	1.7%	0.3%	30.7%	6.3%
Singapore	5,079	5.2%	3.5%	22.5%	4.3%
Slovakia	5,433	4.5%	3.8%	30.6%	15.6%
Slovenia	2,054	2.0%	3.5%	26.8%	21.4%
Solomon Islands	526	16.5%	10.6%	38.4%	15.5%
Somalia	9,636	0.8%	0.5%	19.7%	2.3%
South Africa	51,452	3.3%	0.9%	22.2%	9.0%
South Sudan	9,941	-	-	-	-
Spain	46,182	2.9%	3.4%	29.9%	23.4%
Sri Lanka	20,759	0.3%	0.5%	23.6%	1.0%
State of Palestine	4,013	13.4%	2.2%	41.4%	3.1%
Sudan	35,652	5.8%	2.4%	8.3%	1.0%
Suriname	525	1.3%	0.4%	9.9%	2.3%
Swaziland	1,193	0.8%	0.5%	14.8%	2.7%
Sweden	9,382	1.3%	2.4%	12.7%	15.2%
Switzerland	7,831	2.6%	2.2%	23.4%	19.3%
Syrian Arab Republic	21,533	0.4%	0.4%	28.3%	6.3%
Tajikistan	7,627	0.1%	0.1%	30.0%	2.6%
Tanzania	44,973	0.5%	0.1%	19.9%	1.5%
Thailand	66,402	0.9%	0.1%	37.4%	2.2%
Timor-Leste	1,079	6.4%	1.7%	61.1%	4.3%
Togo	6,306	0.1%	0.5%	13.8%	1.5%
Trinidad and Tobago	1,328	1.0%	0.7%	27.4%	7.1%
Tunisia	10,632	1.3%	0.4%	45.1%	4.4%
Turkey	72,138	3.5%	1.2%	39.2%	13.7%
Turkmenistan	5,042	1.0%	0.3%	36.8%	3.1%
Uganda	33,987	1.0%	1.5%	17.4%	2.0%
Ukraine	46,050	5.6%	2.1%	46.4%	11.9%
United Arab Emirates	8,442	1.4%	0.3%	18.1%	2.5%
United Kingdom	62,066	5.6%	8.7%	23.2%	20.3%
United States of America	312,247	0.4%	0.5%	17.2%	14.2%
Uruguay	3,372	5.7%	8.5%	27.3%	20.4%
Uzbekistan	27,769	0.5%	0.1%	21.7%	1.6%
Vanuatu	236	10.3%	3.8%	28.5%	3.1%
Venezuela	29,043	0.6%	0.3%	21.6%	11.8%
Viet Nam	89,047	0.4%	0.3%	41.2%	1.0%
Western Sahara	515	-	-	-	-
Yemen	22,763	1.0%	0.7%	26.2%	6.8%
Zambia	13,217	1.1%	0.5%	23.9%	3.3%
Zimbabwe	13,077	1.1%	0.1%	24.6%	2.7%

Prevalence (%) of overweight and obesity (BMI>25), 2008		Percentage of one-year-olds* GIVEN THE 3-SERIES HEPATITIS B VACCINATION, 2012	The risk of getting cancer: PROBABILITY OF DEVELOPING A CANCER BEFORE AGE 75, 2012	Countries
Male	Female			
51.7%	45.4%	96%	23.1%	Romania
55.8%	58.9%	97%	21.5%	Russian Federation
24.0%	17.5%	98%	14.4%	Rwanda
82.6%	88.9%	99%	10.3%	Samoa
70.2%	73.2%	98%	9.8%	Saudi Arabia
18.0%	37.0%	92%	10.6%	Senegal
65.3%	46.2%	97%	27.1%	Serbia
21.2%	33.4%	84%	9.5%	Sierra Leone
32.3%	23.7%	96%	20.9%	Singapore
63.9%	53.2%	99%	27.8%	Slovakia
67.6%	55.2%	0%	29.4%	Slovenia
64.9%	71.1%	90%	11.9%	Solomon Islands
18.9%	24.0%	0%	14.7%	Somalia
62.0%	73.6%	73%	19.0%	South Africa
21.6%	28.2%	0%	14.0%	South Sudan
65.1%	50.9%	96%	25.2%	Spain
16.5%	26.5%	99%	10.2%	Sri Lanka
-	-	-	15.3%	State of Palestine
21.6%	28.2%	92%	9.5%	Sudan
51.7%	64.8%	84%	16.5%	Suriname
28.2%	68.2%	95%	10.9%	Swaziland
57.3%	42.5%	0%	27.8%	Sweden
55.0%	34.1%	0%	28.8%	Switzerland
63.4%	69.3%	43%	15.3%	Syrian Arab Republic
33.7%	33.9%	94%	12.7%	Tajikistan
22.1%	25.8%	92%	12.8%	Tanzania
25.8%	36.4%	98%	14.2%	Thailand
10.2%	16.5%	67%	17.6%	Timor-Leste
17.4%	23.3%	84%	9.3%	Togo
59.7%	69.6%	92%	20.7%	Trinidad and Tobago
47.5%	64.2%	97%	11.8%	Tunisia
61.4%	65.8%	96%	21.1%	Turkey
47.1%	40.4%	98%	15.1%	Turkmenistan
22.2%	20.4%	78%	17.6%	Uganda
49.8%	53.2%	46%	20.4%	Ukraine
71.3%	73.9%	94%	10.2%	United Arab Emirates
65.6%	57.5%	0%	26.9%	United Kingdom
72.5%	66.3%	92%	31.1%	United States of America
59.0%	55.4%	95%	25.0%	Uruguay
48.9%	47.2%	99%	10.7%	Uzbekistan
62.4%	68.5%	59%	11.8%	Vanuatu
67.9%	67.0%	81%	15.2%	Venezuela
9.4%	10.8%	97%	14.5%	Viet Nam
-	-	-	10.3%	Western Sahara
40.2%	51.0%	82%	8.4%	Yemen
9.1%	26.0%	78%	13.5%	Zambia
17.6%	40.3%	89%	18.9%	Zimbabwe

*Countries with 0% coverage may represent countries where hepatitis B is not endemic (e.g. Scandinavian countries) and national hepatitis B vaccination programs have not been introduced.

STATISTICS ON CANCER

Countries	Male						Female					
	ALL SITES (excluding nonmelanoma skin cancer)	LUNG	LIVER	ESOPHAGUS	PROSTATE	COLORECTAL	ALL SITES (excluding nonmelanoma skin cancer)	LUNG	BREAST	STOMACH	CERVIX	COLORECTAL
Afghanistan	112.4	10.3	6.6	11.8	3.7	6.0	119.5	3.4	35.1	8.6	8.8	3.6
Albania	185.0	36.5	5.1	1.8	15.8	9.0	173.2	16.6	53.9	15.1	5.0	7.9
Algeria	116.2	17.0	1.7	0.8	8.8	12.1	132.7	3.4	48.5	4.6	8.5	11.0
Angola	89.9	2.9	6.7	6.3	25.0	5.2	112.2	1.3	23.5	3.6	35.5	4.9
Argentina	230.4	32.5	4.4	6.2	44.1	29.8	211.8	11.8	71.2	4.2	20.8	19.1
Armenia	305.6	72.9	14.4	2.2	27.4	22.8	226.4	10.3	74.1	9.1	13.8	17.0
Australia	373.9	33.3	6.4	5.4	115.2	45.5	278.6	21.5	86.0	3.1	5.5	32.0
Austria	295.2	37.1	8.1	5.0	74.7	34.0	222.7	19.5	68.0	4.8	5.8	19.6
Azerbaijan	165.8	20.2	6.4	6.3	8.5	7.1	124.0	4.3	25.4	8.8	9.8	6.4
Bahamas	199.5	16.2	2.7	2.7	74.1	21.1	223.4	4.9	98.9	4.7	20.6	19.9
Bahrain	112.8	21.3	3.6	2.2	13.5	11.8	121.9	8.5	42.5	3.1	5.9	11.0
Bangladesh	109.4	16.6	3.3	15.9	1.7	4.3	100.0	3.6	21.7	4.1	19.2	2.9
Barbados	277.2	8.1	1.8	3.3	123.1	31.7	258.1	2.6	94.7	3.8	25.4	26.1
Belarus	275.5	56.9	3.4	6.8	34.4	30.9	190.6	6.2	45.9	12.2	13.2	20.7
Belgium	364.8	56.6	4.7	7.5	90.9	45.2	288.9	19.9	111.9	3.8	8.6	29.5
Belize	160.6	16.3	7.8	4.1	50.4	9.5	161.2	7.6	39.6	4.1	32.7	8.5
Benin	87.2	2.2	19.2	1.4	25.7	5.2	102.7	0.9	30.2	3.6	27.6	3.7
Bhutan	82.0	6.5	6.1	6.5	1.2	4.7	77.1	7.4	4.6	10.8	12.8	2.0
Bolivia (Plurinational State of)	123.9	5.7	3.7	1.3	25.9	8.9	164.3	4.7	19.2	7.5	47.7	9.3
Bosnia and Herzegovina	180.0	45.2	5.8	1.7	21.4	20.7	147.8	10.9	37.4	6.0	13.7	13.3
Botswana	113.9	8.9	8.0	15.4	12.0	4.3	104.7	1.5	19.9	0.5	30.3	2.8
Brazil	231.6	21.3	6.0	10.1	76.2	16.9	186.8	12.2	59.5	6.0	16.3	14.9
Brunei Darussalam	149.5	24.7	8.7	0.5	21.8	29.9	179.0	22.0	48.6	5.5	16.9	17.4
Bulgaria	260.5	51.6	6.4	3.0	23.5	40.0	220.1	9.0	58.5	7.0	24.5	25.1
Burkina Faso	75.9	3.0	18.5	2.1	19.1	3.1	99.8	2.0	22.7	2.9	23.3	2.0
Burundi	132.2	1.8	6.1	19.0	41.4	5.7	143.0	1.6	23.5	2.8	49.3	6.2
Cambodia	155.3	20.7	32.7	4.2	5.6	10.5	134.1	7.1	19.3	3.3	23.8	6.6
Cameroon	81.2	2.0	7.3	1.5	23.0	3.2	114.1	1.0	35.2	2.0	30.0	3.3
Canada	320.8	42.5	5.5	4.6	88.9	42.6	277.4	34.4	79.8	3.1	6.3	28.5
Cape Verde	60.9	1.5	18.6	0.4	19.0	3.4	88.4	0.2	25.1	3.9	29.0	3.5
Central African Republic	86.9	2.2	7.7	2.9	23.6	5.1	99.7	0.9	31.4	1.6	21.0	3.9
Chad	77.4	1.5	9.3	2.1	18.3	4.6	99.2	0.9	34.1	1.6	18.8	3.8
Chile	195.3	17.1	5.4	4.9	52.4	15.7	163.3	10.2	34.8	9.2	12.8	14.4
China	211.2	52.8	33.7	18.6	5.3	16.9	139.9	20.4	22.1	13.1	7.5	11.6
Colombia	175.2	15.9	3.2	3.0	51.3	13.4	151.5	7.1	35.7	9.0	18.7	12.5
Comoros	81.9	2.6	4.2	12.5	23.2	2.3	121.8	0.0	17.4	0.6	61.3	3.2
Congo	83.7	1.8	9.8	1.5	37.4	6.1	94.1	0.5	31.7	1.7	25.2	5.2
Congo (Democratic Republic of)	102.5	1.6	13.8	5.4	31.1	5.0	115.2	0.6	23.5	5.6	33.1	5.6
Costa Rica	193.5	9.8	5.2	2.0	67.5	17.0	169.2	5.0	45.4	13.7	11.4	15.9
Côte d'Ivoire	78.2	2.0	22.6	1.6	19.6	4.4	101.0	1.4	33.7	2.8	21.7	5.3
Croatia	319.9	58.2	8.1	5.4	46.2	44.2	231.6	15.4	60.0	6.2	10.0	24.7
Cuba	250.8	42.9	4.0	7.7	84.2	17.6	190.3	23.8	50.4	4.4	17.1	21.6
Cyprus	218.2	26.0	3.8	1.6	55.1	27.3	198.2	7.4	78.4	3.3	4.1	22.2
Czech Republic	345.9	50.9	6.4	5.6	72.2	54.0	258.9	17.8	70.3	5.3	14.1	27.1
Denmark	354.3	41.6	4.5	5.6	91.3	45.9	328.8	37.6	105.0	3.1	10.6	35.7
Djibouti	73.7	2.9	4.0	3.8	8.5	7.4	111.3	2.5	35.9	2.3	17.3	5.0

Cancer survivors: Five-year cancer survivors as a proportion (PER 100,000) OF THE COUNTRY'S POPULATION	Estimated cancer mortality rates for all sites (excluding nonmelanoma skin cancer), (AGE-STANDARDIZED RATE [WORLD] PER 100,000 POPULATION), 2012		Countries
	Male	Female	
233.1	103.4	92.9	Afghanistan
723.5	130.9	95.5	Albania
322.7	79.8	70.9	Algeria
206.0	77.0	76.0	Angola
883.8	141.7	96.7	Argentina
868.9	209.6	110.4	Armenia
1929.0	115.4	80.1	Australia
1590.0	129.4	83.1	Austria
363.7	118.7	73.3	Azerbaijan
801.7	118.8	89.6	Bahamas
184.4	60.9	50.6	Bahrain
235.9	89.9	71.9	Bangladesh
1321.4	135.5	93.8	Barbados
966.6	186.0	79.9	Belarus
2142.6	151.0	88.5	Belgium
435.5	106.6	88.6	Belize
207.1	78.1	71.5	Benin
150.8	72.6	62.2	Bhutan
417.4	86.2	96.3	Bolivia (Plurinational State of)
814.1	125.4	71.3	Bosnia and Herzegovina
232.5	85.6	60.4	Botswana
720.2	123.8	87.9	Brazil
378.4	81.3	77.1	Brunei Darussalam
1188.3	160.5	89.5	Bulgaria
164.4	72.1	80.3	Burkina Faso
267.7	125.3	115.2	Burundi
290.7	136.5	95.9	Cambodia
248.6	66.9	73.0	Cameroon
1861.2	117.6	91.7	Canada
199.1	50.0	51.5	Cape Verde
216.0	76.8	73.5	Central African Republic
203.3	71.9	74.8	Chad
660.0	120.4	90.6	Chile
456.0	164.6	82.6	China
501.2	95.7	77.5	Colombia
219.8	75.1	89.4	Comoros
194.8	65.0	56.6	Congo
205.7	96.1	93.4	Congo (Democratic Republic of)
615.1	96.6	75.5	Costa Rica
194.0	69.6	72.1	Côte d'Ivoire
1657.5	190.7	96.4	Croatia
983.8	146.5	104.2	Cuba
1114.8	96.4	62.9	Cyprus
1607.7	158.1	94.2	Czech Republic
2011.2	142.7	110.7	Denmark
208.5	66.7	79.6	Djibouti

STATISTICS ON CANCER

Estimated cancer incidence rates
(AGE-STANDARDIZED RATE [WORLD] PER 100,000 POPULATION), 2012

Countries	Male						Female					
	ALL SITES (excluding nonmelanoma skin cancer)	LUNG	LIVER	ESOPHAGUS	PROSTATE	COLORECTAL	ALL SITES (excluding nonmelanoma skin cancer)	LUNG	BREAST	STOMACH	CERVIX	COLORECTAL
Dominican Republic	158.5	14.9	9.4	1.7	68.5	9.9	149.1	9.2	38.1	6.4	30.7	10.5
Ecuador	162.0	9.1	4.9	1.5	54.4	10.0	169.2	5.6	32.7	13.4	29.0	11.3
Egypt	158.4	11.2	38.1	2.8	7.8	6.1	147.8	3.8	49.5	2.3	2.3	5.2
El Salvador	136.6	7.2	7.2	2.1	27.0	7.9	167.2	4.9	23.7	14.1	24.8	8.9
Equatorial Guinea	76.1	5.9	5.1	2.2	19.4	4.6	98.5	1.7	25.2	2.0	25.1	4.0
Eritrea	82.8	3.0	4.1	4.1	8.5	7.5	118.6	2.2	35.9	2.0	17.4	5.0
Estonia	321.9	48.2	3.4	4.5	94.4	35.1	202.7	9.4	51.6	10.3	19.9	22.6
Ethiopia	73.2	3.3	1.8	2.0	6.4	8.5	140.9	3.1	41.8	2.9	26.4	6.3
Fiji	91.3	7.2	12.0	3.0	17.3	6.9	189.3	4.9	65.0	3.0	37.8	7.3
Finland	290.1	29.9	7.4	3.7	96.6	28.2	234.2	12.2	89.4	3.9	4.3	19.7
France	385.3	52.0	11.3	6.1	127.3	36.1	276.7	20.2	104.5	2.8	6.8	24.9
French Guiana	174.1	10.2	6.2	6.1	40.6	7.0	150.1	4.5	37.1	4.3	36.6	2.8
French Polynesia	287.4	53.3	7.1	5.6	114.6	16.1	227.3	21.1	92.2	5.6	8.2	10.6
Gabon	79.9	8.3	2.6	3.0	15.8	5.6	101.5	4.4	16.1	1.7	19.9	4.8
Gambia	67.3	3.5	36.3	1.1	6.7	1.5	69.6	1.2	9.8	0.8	26.1	1.0
Georgia	207.8	30.8	8.5	1.0	18.6	9.9	163.7	4.8	44.0	7.0	14.2	7.5
Germany	323.7	38.8	7.2	6.9	77.3	39.7	252.5	17.9	91.6	5.4	8.2	23.3
Ghana	79.2	3.8	17.6	0.8	13.0	5.4	104.8	1.0	25.6	1.8	35.4	2.9
Greece	194.8	50.9	5.3	1.6	20.2	16.3	138.0	9.0	43.9	3.6	5.2	11.2
Greenland	-	-	-	-	-	-	-	-	-	-	-	-
Guadeloupe	260.9	14.7	5.6	5.8	105.2	16.9	163.8	6.2	53.7	7.0	13.0	11.6
Guam	198.0	47.6	12.0	2.9	60.0	25.1	143.0	22.7	49.4	0.0	9.0	16.4
Guatemala	116.4	7.9	16.0	2.1	22.3	4.2	142.7	5.2	11.9	23.4	22.3	4.4
Guinea	88.9	2.0	25.3	0.8	34.7	2.4	94.0	0.9	14.5	2.7	38.4	1.3
Guinea-Bissau	70.0	2.0	18.5	0.8	19.0	3.8	96.0	1.3	26.0	2.6	29.8	3.1
Guyana	144.4	6.1	7.7	2.5	65.8	9.8	193.5	2.7	50.4	2.3	46.9	9.0
Haiti	102.9	7.3	7.6	2.3	38.6	6.0	111.5	6.9	22.0	6.4	24.9	7.7
Honduras	116.0	7.9	11.3	2.0	22.7	6.5	146.7	4.9	19.9	15.3	29.4	7.1
Hungary	356.1	76.6	5.6	6.9	37.5	58.9	236.5	33.2	54.5	6.5	18.0	30.5
Iceland	299.5	31.0	2.1	6.7	106.6	28.9	274.2	28.9	96.3	3.7	7.9	28.2
India	92.4	11.0	3.5	5.4	4.2	7.2	97.4	3.1	25.8	3.7	22.0	5.1
Indonesia	136.2	25.8	13.4	1.5	14.8	15.9	134.4	8.1	40.3	1.9	17.3	10.1
Iran (Islamic Republic of)	134.7	10.3	2.8	9.0	12.6	11.6	120.1	5.0	28.1	9.7	2.8	10.5
Iraq	144.6	24.2	4.4	1.4	8.7	7.9	131.7	6.6	42.6	4.4	2.8	6.5
Ireland	343.3	36.1	4.5	8.4	114.2	43.1	278.9	27.4	92.3	4.4	13.6	27.7
Israel	318.0	29.5	3.4	1.7	84.3	43.0	258.7	14.4	80.5	4.9	4.6	30.3
Italy	312.9	38.5	11.0	2.1	67.6	41.5	255.2	13.2	91.3	5.9	6.7	27.5
Jamaica	222.0	29.8	5.8	3.8	88.0	15.2	179.2	7.6	55.8	6.1	26.3	13.7
Japan	260.4	38.8	14.6	11.1	30.4	42.1	185.7	12.9	51.5	16.5	10.9	23.5
Jordan	153.3	27.0	5.4	1.2	15.3	29.8	157.8	4.1	61.0	5.3	2.4	21.2
Kazakhstan	282.2	59.2	12.2	15.8	14.9	29.1	216.7	8.1	63.0	12.8	29.4	19.4
Kenya	167.2	3.4	6.4	20.5	31.6	10.3	196.6	2.0	38.3	8.4	40.1	7.2
Korea (Democratic People's Republic of)	204.2	58.5	25.8	9.5	3.2	26.7	170.0	33.4	50.0	0.0	20.1	10.0
Korea (Republic of)	340.0	45.5	36.7	6.0	30.3	58.7	293.6	16.2	52.1	24.7	9.5	33.3
Kuwait	89.8	9.9	5.3	0.7	14.5	12.6	123.3	4.9	46.7	2.1	4.0	13.3
Kyrgyzstan	151.6	26.9	11.0	6.9	7.3	8.1	129.4	6.7	27.3	10.3	23.7	8.3
Lao People's Democratic Republic	165.5	20.6	78.7	0.9	3.5	10.1	122.4	6.9	19.0	1.7	12.5	7.7

Cancer survivors: Five-year cancer survivors as a proportion (PER 100,000) OF THE COUNTRY'S POPULATION	Estimated cancer mortality rates for all sites (excluding nonmelanoma skin cancer), (AGE-STANDARDIZED RATE [WORLD] PER 100,000 POPULATION), 2012		Countries
	Male	**Female**	**Countries**
503.8	100.5	81.4	Dominican Republic
534.3	96.2	94.2	Ecuador
372.2	120.5	88.7	Egypt
470.8	91.9	97.8	El Salvador
224.4	67.6	65.0	Equatorial Guinea
201.7	76.3	90.7	Eritrea
1312.3	159.3	72.9	Estonia
250.9	64.9	103.1	Ethiopia
451.7	65.5	104.3	Fiji
1853.6	104.9	72.1	Finland
2165.5	143.4	79.0	France
524.2	118.5	76.3	French Guiana
806.2	153.8	116.3	French Polynesia
207.3	54.9	55.4	Gabon
82.8	62.6	54.2	Gambia
687.7	127.4	77.2	Georgia
1964.6	122.1	83.4	Germany
211.7	63.8	64.0	Ghana
1046.6	132.2	70.6	Greece
-	-	-	Greenland
1059.1	124.6	70.1	Guadeloupe
531.0	105.5	54.7	Guam
316.2	93.0	99.5	Guatemala
178.0	79.9	71.0	Guinea
183.6	64.4	71.4	Guinea-Bissau
517.2	110.0	103.2	Guyana
281.8	88.4	80.3	Haiti
331.8	89.3	92.2	Honduras
1333.5	208.2	112.4	Hungary
1749.0	99.3	78.4	Iceland
202.9	69.7	60.2	India
357.7	103.8	78.5	Indonesia
290.1	90.4	72.7	Iran (Islamic Republic of)
274.3	113.0	86.7	Iraq
1528.5	123.3	96.4	Ireland
1445.8	108.0	84.1	Israel
1933.8	128.6	81.3	Italy
716.9	133.5	87.6	Jamaica
1830.7	125.1	69.2	Japan
337.4	105.2	85.5	Jordan
668.8	202.5	104.8	Kazakhstan
335.1	139.1	133.3	Kenya
480.4	155.5	105.7	Korea (Democratic People's Republic of)
1522.7	145.7	65.4	Korea (Republic of)
234.0	46.4	69.3	Kuwait
300.6	125.2	81.2	Kyrgyzstan
226.3	148.8	92.2	Lao People's Democratic Republic

STATISTICS ON CANCER

Estimated cancer incidence rates
(AGE-STANDARDIZED RATE [WORLD] PER 100,000 POPULATION), 2012

Countries	Male						Female					
	ALL SITES (excluding nonmelanoma skin cancer)	LUNG	LIVER	ESOPHAGUS	PROSTATE	COLORECTAL	ALL SITES (excluding nonmelanoma skin cancer)	LUNG	BREAST	STOMACH	CERVIX	COLORECTAL
Latvia	325.0	58.0	5.6	7.1	82.7	30.0	206.5	7.9	52.1	8.7	17.3	20.2
Lebanon	203.9	30.2	3.3	0.9	37.2	19.1	192.8	11.0	78.7	4.7	4.6	13.5
Lesotho	114.0	5.3	10.7	21.0	12.1	3.0	96.7	1.1	9.0	0.8	38.4	1.2
Liberia	82.9	1.9	24.0	1.2	27.2	3.1	97.0	1.1	24.1	2.8	30.1	3.2
Libya	135.9	28.0	5.4	1.6	15.5	14.5	113.1	3.7	24.1	2.8	9.7	14.3
Lithuania	311.8	55.4	4.7	7.6	60.9	31.2	224.0	7.2	48.7	8.0	26.1	18.9
Luxembourg	309.1	39.9	10.3	6.4	78.8	42.1	259.6	18.5	89.1	5.2	4.9	21.6
Macedonia (The former Yugoslav Republic of)	265.5	71.3	5.7	1.2	27.6	28.4	220.8	13.7	76.2	10.6	12.4	20.5
Madagascar	142.4	12.5	5.0	11.3	32.9	9.0	134.3	2.4	26.6	3.0	44.6	7.1
Malawi	123.5	1.2	1.8	28.2	10.8	3.4	186.4	0.7	16.8	2.5	75.9	3.4
Malaysia	144.9	26.9	8.7	2.5	10.8	21.1	143.4	9.2	38.7	5.7	15.6	15.7
Maldives	91.6	13.2	5.3	6.0	6.4	6.6	84.8	1.8	31.6	0.7	11.0	4.9
Mali	83.8	3.8	7.5	1.5	12.8	6.2	135.6	1.9	29.8	8.2	44.2	5.9
Malta	267.7	36.5	3.6	3.7	50.8	39.9	228.9	7.7	85.9	5.5	3.8	25.2
Martinique	358.4	13.0	3.7	4.5	227.2	25.3	157.4	6.3	59.6	5.8	8.7	23.1
Mauritania	74.4	2.0	18.9	1.2	19.0	3.9	97.7	0.9	25.8	2.9	29.4	3.3
Mauritius	171.1	16.3	2.3	4.6	22.9	22.3	193.9	5.3	64.2	5.8	15.0	15.8
Mexico	123.9	10.5	5.9	1.6	27.3	8.9	139.9	4.9	35.4	6.0	23.3	6.7
Moldova (Republic of)	230.0	43.3	12.5	3.4	19.7	36.0	170.2	8.3	38.7	6.5	19.6	23.0
Mongolia	237.7	27.7	97.8	21.2	3.4	5.7	171.9	5.8	9.4	20.2	24.3	6.3
Montenegro	262.7	62.4	7.0	2.8	33.7	36.2	219.7	19.3	59.7	7.0	20.2	21.1
Morocco	122.7	25.5	1.5	1.6	18.5	9.9	114.4	2.8	40.8	3.0	14.3	7.3
Mozambique	118.3	4.2	6.3	12.5	9.6	1.5	153.0	1.8	14.5	0.5	65.0	1.0
Myanmar	149.4	25.0	16.1	11.4	4.3	10.3	134.6	16.2	22.1	7.7	20.6	7.4
Namibia	86.3	4.9	2.6	2.3	22.2	5.1	81.5	2.1	24.4	1.3	14.7	4.5
Nepal	85.6	14.8	1.2	3.6	1.5	3.8	85.6	10.4	13.7	3.8	19.0	2.7
Netherlands	327.8	44.4	2.4	10.0	83.4	47.5	289.6	31.6	99.0	3.9	6.8	33.9
New Caledonia	330.7	57.0	12.8	5.5	114.9	28.7	269.3	23.6	87.6	4.9	15.3	19.7
New Zealand	320.1	29.2	6.0	5.6	92.2	41.5	274.3	23.2	85.0	3.8	5.3	33.5
Nicaragua	106.1	9.2	11.2	1.8	23.3	7.4	123.1	5.2	23.9	8.5	36.2	8.2
Niger	56.7	0.4	8.8	1.2	9.0	5.0	71.0	0.0	23.8	1.5	8.6	4.6
Nigeria	79.0	1.1	15.0	0.3	30.7	4.5	121.7	1.1	50.4	2.0	29.0	4.0
Norway	368.7	34.8	2.9	3.9	129.7	42.6	277.1	26.1	73.1	3.8	9.8	35.8
Oman	78.6	6.7	4.6	1.8	10.2	7.4	92.4	2.8	26.0	3.9	5.3	7.6
Pakistan	96.0	9.8	4.7	3.9	5.3	4.7	127.7	1.7	50.3	2.2	7.9	3.3
Panama	150.1	12.7	5.6	2.4	39.4	14.1	148.8	5.6	43.0	7.5	18.7	11.1
Papua New Guinea	156.7	11.9	14.9	4.0	16.4	11.1	179.8	4.8	33.7	5.8	34.5	5.6
Paraguay	143.2	23.2	3.0	4.6	34.8	12.9	153.0	5.3	43.8	4.1	34.2	11.3
Peru	140.9	11.3	6.0	1.9	30.4	10.2	169.8	9.1	28.0	15.0	32.7	11.9
Philippines	139.9	31.3	17.1	1.8	18.0	15.6	143.4	9.5	47.0	2.9	16.0	11.0
Poland	269.2	60.5	3.8	4.0	35.9	37.2	205.6	21.8	51.9	4.9	12.2	19.5
Portugal	306.3	34.2	8.6	6.1	63.6	41.8	198.1	8.3	67.0	8.5	0.0	17.1
Puerto Rico	237.2	13.0	7.2	3.4	93.2	29.6	193.5	6.3	57.5	3.1	11.4	20.6
Qatar	104.0	13.4	8.9	1.8	13.2	11.6	134.5	4.1	46.1	5.6	5.1	15.5
Reunion	242.5	32.3	5.8	8.3	54.4	22.0	142.1	4.9	46.6	6.1	15.3	14.6

Cancer survivors: Five-year cancer survivors as a proportion (PER 100,000) OF THE COUNTRY'S POPULATION	Estimated cancer mortality rates for all sites (excluding nonmelanoma skin cancer), (AGE-STANDARDIZED RATE [WORLD] PER 100,000 POPULATION), 2012		Countries
	Male	Female	
1276.5	185.0	96.1	Latvia
633.0	119.5	89.6	Lebanon
197.2	95.0	67.1	Lesotho
172.2	78.1	76.0	Liberia
282.4	88.9	62.2	Libya
1239.5	194.9	88.8	Lithuania
1914.0	117.2	80.6	Luxembourg
1185.0	183.9	106.5	Macedonia (The former Yugoslav Republic of)
288.5	117.2	92.0	Madagascar
341.7	110.7	137.8	Malawi
384.1	91.8	80.2	Malaysia
212.0	63.8	42.3	Maldives
231.2	77.3	101.4	Mali
1451.2	109.0	75.0	Malta
1439.8	120.8	76.4	Martinique
178.2	68.3	68.2	Mauritania
530.2	127.2	84.3	Mauritius
430.2	72.2	66.9	Mexico
787.7	163.6	88.4	Moldova (Republic of)
260.9	202.5	127.2	Mongolia
1116.9	174.8	108.8	Montenegro
336.1	92.3	66.8	Morocco
308.3	108.6	121.4	Mozambique
322.9	128.9	99.8	Myanmar
197.4	61.2	45.5	Namibia
187.6	72.6	64.1	Nepal
1939.8	136.5	102.4	Netherlands
1004.9	146.0	112.0	New Caledonia
1759.5	114.4	95.4	New Zealand
301.1	83.4	79.6	Nicaragua
151.2	53.7	55.2	Niger
243.6	67.4	78.0	Nigeria
2020.1	114.3	88.4	Norway
143.1	57.8	54.0	Oman
291.8	75.4	83.6	Pakistan
498.0	88.8	71.1	Panama
385.2	131.7	124.5	Papua New Guinea
446.9	101.3	83.5	Paraguay
462.7	92.0	93.5	Peru
340.2	107.4	78.6	Philippines
1072.1	176.0	100.0	Poland
1473.9	134.7	70.1	Portugal
1017.4	89.3	57.6	Puerto Rico
175.7	71.8	66.6	Qatar
589.0	116.8	52.7	Reunion

STATISTICS ON CANCER

Estimated cancer incidence rates
(AGE-STANDARDIZED RATE [WORLD] PER 100,000 POPULATION), 2012

Countries	Male						Female					
	ALL SITES (excluding nonmelanoma skin cancer)	LUNG	LIVER	ESOPHAGUS	PROSTATE	COLORECTAL	ALL SITES (excluding nonmelanoma skin cancer)	LUNG	BREAST	STOMACH	CERVIX	COLORECTAL
Romania	271.0	58.8	9.2	4.3	24.2	34.5	190.6	11.2	50.0	5.8	28.6	20.2
Russian Federation	245.8	51.4	4.4	6.4	30.1	30.0	187.1	6.8	45.6	10.8	15.3	21.8
Rwanda	130.2	1.6	18.6	9.4	25.6	3.9	142.3	0.8	15.9	9.7	41.8	6.1
Samoa	92.5	9.4	5.0	0.0	10.9	9.0	96.1	0.0	23.2	5.8	17.1	4.2
Saudi Arabia	85.9	7.3	6.4	1.4	9.5	12.6	102.8	2.7	29.5	2.4	2.7	10.8
Senegal	85.5	2.9	16.5	1.2	23.6	4.2	115.0	1.4	22.4	5.5	41.4	3.6
Serbia	299.2	70.3	6.6	4.1	36.6	43.4	247.6	23.9	69.0	5.7	23.8	23.3
Sierra Leone	83.8	1.9	23.8	1.3	27.2	3.4	97.7	1.3	24.3	2.7	30.2	3.3
Singapore	218.8	35.7	15.8	2.9	33.1	40.1	198.7	15.5	65.7	5.8	8.1	28.0
Slovakia	338.2	47.5	6.8	6.4	50.0	61.6	238.0	14.3	57.5	6.6	16.1	29.3
Slovenia	358.2	53.8	8.4	3.7	82.9	49.7	251.5	17.5	66.5	6.4	10.5	27.0
Solomon Islands	89.3	12.4	17.3	0.3	11.3	6.1	145.2	3.1	47.6	2.0	28.5	7.9
Somalia	111.9	3.3	4.1	11.3	19.0	9.4	165.2	2.5	40.6	5.7	33.4	6.8
South Africa	224.3	28.7	6.5	13.9	67.9	15.6	168.9	11.2	41.5	3.1	31.7	9.5
South Sudan	123.1	2.7	7.5	11.7	25.5	7.5	143.0	1.9	31.8	4.2	30.4	5.8
Spain	312.8	52.5	9.9	4.5	65.2	43.9	198.2	11.3	67.3	5.1	7.8	24.2
Sri Lanka	86.9	9.8	4.4	5.7	3.0	3.9	102.7	3.2	30.9	5.2	13.1	3.5
State of Palestine	150.5	21.3	5.1	2.3	15.2	15.9	142.7	5.2	44.0	5.2	2.0	15.0
Sudan	92.0	2.7	6.5	5.8	10.3	6.1	91.0	1.3	27.8	0.9	7.9	3.2
Suriname	163.8	20.1	8.5	1.1	37.9	23.0	162.7	6.9	41.4	3.2	38.0	12.1
Swaziland	122.1	5.4	18.6	9.6	17.4	3.2	111.9	1.4	10.5	1.3	53.1	1.6
Sweden	296.8	19.4	3.4	3.5	119.0	32.3	248.7	19.1	80.4	2.7	7.4	26.5
Switzerland	337.9	35.1	8.7	6.1	107.2	36.3	245.9	20.7	83.1	3.6	3.6	23.6
Syrian Arab Republic	148.3	25.5	4.9	1.3	11.9	18.8	145.2	5.3	52.5	4.8	2.6	13.8
Tajikistan	128.7	10.9	8.5	19.8	2.3	7.3	112.3	5.1	20.4	15.0	9.9	4.0
Tanzania	115.8	0.9	2.9	12.9	34.6	3.8	132.7	0.5	19.4	2.6	54.0	5.8
Thailand	149.6	30.7	34.8	4.4	7.2	15.2	128.8	12.6	29.3	2.5	17.8	10.1
Timor-Leste	183.9	43.8	11.1	2.6	16.5	18.1	149.6	19.1	32.6	1.9	13.3	9.1
Togo	77.2	2.2	15.8	4.1	14.6	4.6	104.8	0.8	27.2	5.0	21.5	3.0
Trinidad and Tobago	273.5	22.7	2.9	2.2	123.9	33.4	180.3	4.8	56.9	2.4	24.5	16.8
Tunisia	127.0	31.1	1.4	0.6	11.3	11.9	95.7	1.7	31.8	3.2	4.8	10.0
Turkey	257.8	63.9	4.7	4.3	40.6	20.5	161.6	8.8	39.1	10.9	4.3	13.1
Turkmenistan	159.4	21.3	8.8	24.0	2.1	9.3	132.8	5.6	26.8	13.6	13.1	9.0
Uganda	175.7	2.7	9.2	24.8	48.2	7.7	167.4	2.7	27.5	3.0	44.4	6.6
Ukraine	231.9	46.9	3.0	5.5	20.3	29.9	174.7	6.1	41.3	9.1	16.6	19.8
United Arab Emirates	83.8	11.2	3.5	1.8	10.0	8.6	127.1	5.2	39.2	3.4	9.5	8.7
United Kingdom	284.0	34.9	4.6	10.0	73.2	36.8	267.3	25.9	95.0	3.1	7.1	24.4
United States of America	347.0	44.2	9.8	5.5	98.2	28.5	297.4	33.7	92.9	2.7	6.6	22.0
Uruguay	297.5	50.7	2.9	8.8	60.6	35.0	220.9	9.2	69.8	6.7	18.9	25.4
Uzbekistan	96.9	13.1	6.3	7.2	2.0	5.6	103.5	3.7	27.1	8.8	13.5	4.9
Vanuatu	98.2	16.6	23.6	0.0	4.7	5.4	117.0	2.3	31.8	3.9	19.2	7.5
Venezuela	146.9	20.6	4.3	2.0	35.8	11.5	155.0	11.8	41.2	6.2	32.8	9.8
Viet Nam	172.9	41.1	40.2	5.8	3.4	11.5	114.2	12.2	23.0	10.2	10.6	9.0
Western Sahara	89.0	14.8	4.4	0.4	16.2	7.7	107.8	0.9	36.2	5.7	31.1	5.9
Yemen	81.2	6.4	4.1	4.4	2.7	5.9	80.7	1.7	27.4	2.5	3.1	3.2
Zambia	115.1	2.4	3.6	11.0	21.9	5.2	157.8	1.4	22.4	4.0	58.0	4.5
Zimbabwe	167.0	7.2	8.0	11.8	37.3	8.1	209.1	3.2	28.5	8.0	56.4	9.3

Cancer survivors: **Five-year cancer survivors as a proportion** (PER 100,000) OF THE COUNTRY'S POPULATION	**Estimated cancer mortality rates for all sites (excluding nonmelanoma skin cancer),** (AGE-STANDARDIZED RATE [WORLD] PER 100,000 POPULATION), 2012		**Countries**
	Male	**Female**	
983.7	175.3	89.2	Romania
903.0	176.3	91.3	Russian Federation
255.1	114.0	104.6	Rwanda
254.8	64.4	49.4	Samoa
192.8	56.8	52.7	Saudi Arabia
194.1	76.0	80.8	Senegal
1409.7	186.7	115.2	Serbia
166.8	82.2	78.4	Sierra Leone
843.2	107.6	75.9	Singapore
1207.8	173.4	92.5	Slovakia
1648.8	167.7	93.9	Slovenia
310.9	77.9	94.6	Solomon Islands
299.1	96.0	116.7	Somalia
464.3	144.1	103.3	South Africa
297.2	108.4	106.0	South Sudan
1467.6	136.1	67.0	Spain
321.9	56.8	52.8	Sri Lanka
306.8	113.8	89.1	State of Palestine
198.8	80.1	67.0	Sudan
532.3	113.8	87.7	Suriname
238.3	101.9	73.0	Swaziland
1978.0	101.7	85.7	Sweden
1938.9	112.6	77.0	Switzerland
344.9	108.9	87.0	Syrian Arab Republic
232.5	107.6	75.4	Tajikistan
269.4	96.9	89.3	Tanzania
514.9	113.9	77.4	Thailand
322.1	155.6	106.4	Timor-Leste
195.8	68.3	74.8	Togo
789.5	156.0	92.3	Trinidad and Tobago
310.1	84.1	49.3	Tunisia
553.5	179.0	86.7	Turkey
306.8	123.8	84.8	Turkmenistan
307.6	152.7	120.3	Uganda
870.9	160.9	85.0	Ukraine
131.1	57.9	64.9	United Arab Emirates
1594.0	126.0	97.3	United Kingdom
1892.1	123.9	91.7	United States of America
1163.6	197.3	106.5	Uruguay
230.4	77.4	63.4	Uzbekistan
296.2	87.9	66.6	Vanuatu
484.5	95.3	77.9	Venezuela
306.4	148.0	76.3	Viet Nam
244.3	71.7	60.7	Western Sahara
153.7	70.8	59.6	Yemen
286.8	100.5	110.8	Zambia
373.7	138.2	146.5	Zimbabwe

CANCER ATLAS GLOSSARY

Aflatoxin:
A harmful, cancer-causing chemical made by certain types of Aspergillus mold that may be found on poorly stored grains and nuts. Consumption of foods contaminated with aflatoxin is an important risk factor for hepatocellular (liver) cancer.

Age-specific rate:
A rate for a specified age group, in which the numerator and denominator refer to the same age group.

Age-standardization:
A technique that allows comparison of incidence (or mortality) rates between populations, adjusting for any differences in their respective age distributions.

Asbestos:
A natural material that is made of tiny fibers and used in insulation and as a fire retardant. Asbestos exposure is an important risk factor for cancer, especially mesothelioma (lining of the chest, abdomen, and heart) and also lung cancer.

Benign tumor:
An abnormal growth that is not cancer and does not spread to other areas of the body.

Beta-naphthylamine:
A synthetic organic compound formerly used as an intermediate in some manufacturing processes, and an important risk factor for bladder cancer. Its production and commercial use, with the exception of limited laboratory use, has been banned in most countries.

Body mass index (BMI):
A measure of a person's weight in relation to his or her height, calculated as weight in kilograms divided by height in meters squared.

Cancer:
A disease in which abnormal cells divide uncontrollably. Cancer cells can invade nearby tissues and spread through the bloodstream and lymphatic system to other parts of the body.

Cancer registry:
An institution that performs the systematic collection and maintenance of a file or register of all cancer cases occurring in a defined population. Registries continuously and systematically collect information from various data sources on the personal characteristics of cancer patients (e.g. age, sex, and race) and the clinical and pathological characteristics (e.g. stage, histologic classification) of the cancers.

Cancer screening programs:
Programs organized at a national or regional level that aim to decrease the incidence and mortality of a specific type of cancer by identifying precancerous lesions or tumors at an early stage, when they can be effectively treated. Programs usually have: 1) an explicit policy; 2) a team responsible for organizing the screening and delivering appropriate healthcare; and 3) a structure for assuring quality screening and follow-up of abnormal screening tests.

Carcinogen:
Any agent —chemical, physical or biological— that causes cancer. Examples include tobacco smoke, asbestos, human papillomavirus (HPV), and ultraviolet (UV) radiation.

Carcinoma:
A cancerous tumor that begins in the lining layer (epithelial cells) of organs. At least 80% of all cancers are carcinomas.

Chemotherapy:
Treatment with a drug or drugs to destroy cancer cells. Chemotherapy may be used, either alone or in combination with surgery or radiation treatment, to treat cancer when it is at an early stage, when the cancer has spread, when the cancer has come back (recurred), or when there is a strong chance that the cancer could recur.

Colonoscopy:
Examination of the large bowel with a long, flexible, lighted tube called a colonoscope. The physician looks for polyps or early cancers during the exam, and removes them using a wire passed through the colonoscope.

Computerized tomography (CT):
A series of detailed pictures of areas inside the body taken from different angles; the pictures are created by a computer linked to an x-ray machine. Also called computerized axial tomography (CAT) scan. A special kind of CT machine, the spiral CT, has been used to look for early lung cancer.

Diagnosis:
The process of identifying a disease by its signs and symptoms, as well as medical tests and tissue sampling and examination as needed.

Dioxins:
Organic chemical byproducts of industrial processes; considered highly toxic environmental pollutants due to their effects on the immune and endocrine systems and on encouraging tumor growth.

Direct costs:
Expenditures for medical procedures and services associated with the treatment and care of people with cancer.

Disability-adjusted life year (DALY):
A measurement of the years of healthy life lost due to disease in a population. DALYs are the sum of two components: the years of life lost due to premature death, and the years of life lost due to disability.

Electron accelerator machines:
Used in medical radiation therapy, these machines accelerate tiny charged particles called electrons, and deliver uniform doses of high-energy x-rays to the region of the patient's tumor. These x-rays can destroy the cancer cells while sparing the surrounding normal tissue.

Endometrial cancer:
Cancer of the layer of tissue that lines the uterus.

Epidemic:
Occurrence of an illness, condition, or behavior that affects many people in the same region during a specified period of time. To constitute an epidemic, this occurrence must exceed normal occurrence of the disease in the region.

Fecal occult blood test (FOBT):
A test used to screen for large bowel cancer. It looks for blood in the stools, the presence of which may be a sign of cancer.

Helicobacter pylori (H. pylori):
A type of bacterium that causes inflammation and ulcers in the stomach or small intestine. People with *H. pylori* infections may be more likely to develop cancer in the stomach.

Hematopoietic system:
Organs and tissues involved in the production of blood, including the bone marrow, lymph nodes, spleen, and tonsils.

Hepatitis B and C viruses (HBV and HCV):
Viruses that cause hepatitis, a condition that is characterized by inflammation of the liver. Long-term infection may lead to cirrhosis (scarring of the liver) and liver cancer. Persons infected with HCV may also have an increased risk for certain types of non-Hodgkin lymphoma.

Hepatocellular carcinoma:
The most common type of cancer originating in the liver.

High-/middle-/low-income country:
For the 2014 fiscal year, according to the World Bank, a high-income country has a gross national income (GNI) per capita of more than US$12,616; a middle-income country between US$1035 and US$12,616; and a low-income country less than US$1035.

Hormone replacement therapy (HRT):
Hormones (estrogen, progesterone, or other types) given to women after menopause to replace the hormones no longer produced by the ovaries. HRT can be a risk factor for cancers of the endometrium and breast.

Human development index (HDI):
A measure of health, education and income at the country level produced by the United Nations Development Programme as an alternative to purely economic assessments of national progress, such as GDP growth.

Human herpesvirus 8 (HHV-8):
A type of virus that causes Kaposi sarcoma. Patients with acquired immunodeficiency syndrome frequently suffer from HHV-8-associated diseases. Infection with HHV-8 can also cause certain types of lymphoma and severe lymph node enlargement, known as Castleman's disease. HHV-8 is also known as Kaposi sarcoma-associated herpesvirus, or KSHV.

Human immunodeficiency virus (HIV):
The virus that causes acquired immune deficiency syndrome (AIDS). It is transmitted through blood and other body fluids, and infants born to infected mothers may also become infected. Infection with both HIV and HHV-8 increases the risk of developing Kaposi sarcoma.

Human papillomavirus (HPV):
A type of virus that can cause abnormal tissue growth (for example, warts) and other changes to cells. Long-term infection with certain types of human papillomavirus (e.g. types 16 and 18) can cause cervical cancer. HPV is also a risk factor for anal, vaginal, vulvar, penile, oropharyngeal, and squamous cell skin cancers. It is transmitted through sexual contact.

Incidence:
The number of new cases arising in a given period in a specified population. This information, collected routinely by cancer registries, can be expressed as an absolute number of cases per year or as a rate per 100,000 persons per year.

Kaposi sarcoma:
A type of cancer characterized by the abnormal growth of blood vessels that develop into lesions on the skin, lymph nodes, lining of the mouth, nose, and throat, and other tissues of the body. It is caused by human herpesvirus-8 (HHV-8). The risk of developing Kaposi sarcoma in a person who has HHV-8 increases significantly if the person is also infected with human immunodeficiency virus (HIV).

Keratinocyte (nonmelanoma) skin cancer:
Also known as basal or squamous cell skin cancer. A cancer that occurs in keratinocyte cells, which are located in the epidermis (top layer of skin) and are responsible for producing keratin. Keratinocytes are divided into squamous cells on the surface of the epidermis and basal cells located within the deeper basal layer of the epidermis.

Leukemia:
A cancer of the blood or blood-forming organs.

Lumpectomy:
Surgery to remove a breast lump or tumor and a small amount of surrounding normal tissue.

Lymphoma:
A cancer of the lymphatic system. The lymphatic system is a network of thin vessels and nodes throughout the body. The two main types of lymphoma are Hodgkin lymphoma (or disease) and non-Hodgkin lymphoma.

Malignant tumor:
A mass of cancer cells that may invade surrounding tissues or spread (metastasize) to distant areas of the body. Synonymous with cancer.

Mastectomy:
Surgery to remove the entire breast. There are different types of mastectomy that differ in the amount of tissue and lymph nodes removed.

Melanoma:
A cancerous (malignant) tumor that begins in the cells that produce the skin coloring (melanocytes). Melanoma is almost always curable in its early stages. However, it is likely to spread, and once it has spread to other parts of the body the likelihood of cure decreases.

Menarche:
The first menstrual period, usually occurring during puberty.

Menopause:
The time period marked by the permanent cessation of menstruation, usually occurring between the ages of 45 and 55 years.

Mesothelioma:
A benign (not cancer) or malignant (cancer) tumor affecting the lining of the chest or abdomen. Exposure to asbestos particles in the air increases the risk of developing malignant mesothelioma, which is extremely lethal.

Metastasis:
The distant spread of cancer from its primary site to other places in the body.

Morbidity:
Any departure from physiological or psychological well-being. Measures of morbidity for people living with cancer may include disability, pain, time away from work, or days spent in the hospital.

Mortality:
The number of deaths occurring in a given period in a specified population. It can be expressed as an absolute number of deaths per year or as a rate per 100,000 persons per year.

Neoplasm:
An abnormal growth (tumor) that starts from a single altered cell; a neoplasm may be benign or malignant. Cancer is a malignant neoplasm.

Neuroblastoma:
Cancer that arises in immature nerve cells; affects mostly infants and children.

Overweight/obese:
Persons who are considered overweight have a body mass index (BMI) greater than 25; a BMI greater than 30 is considered obese.

Particulate matter:
Microscopic solid or liquid particles associated with the atmosphere that can penetrate the lungs and cause damage that can lead to lung cancer. Particulate matter can be naturally occurring (e.g. originating from volcanoes or dust storms) or synthetic (e.g. vehicle emissions). The smallest class of particulate matter (<2.5 micrometers diameter) is the deadliest.

Palliative care:
An approach that aims to improve the quality of life for patients and families facing the problems associated with life-threatening cancers. It provides for prevention and relief of suffering through treatment for pain and other symptoms as well as through spiritual and psychosocial support, at the time of cancer diagnosis, through the end of life, and during family bereavement.

Prevalence:
The number of persons in a defined population who have been diagnosed with a specific type of cancer, and who are still alive at the end of a given year (the survivors). Five-year prevalence limits the number of patients to those diagnosed in the past 5 years. It is a particularly useful measure of cancer burden because for most cancers, patients who are still alive five years after diagnosis are usually considered cured. However, exceptions to this include breast cancer patients, who continue to die from the disease 5 years after diagnosis.

Prognosis:
Prediction of the course of cancer, and the outlook for a cure of the cancer.

Radiotherapy:
The use of radiation treatment to kill cancer cells or stop them from dividing.

Radon:
A radioactive gas that is released by uranium—a substance found in soil and rock—and is an important risk factor for lung cancer.

Rate:
see Incidence and Mortality.

Retinoblastoma:
A rare form of eye cancer that affects the retina of infants and young children.

Sarcoma:
A cancer of the bone, cartilage, fat, muscle, blood vessels, or other connective or supportive tissue.

Sigmoidoscopy:
An examination to help find cancer or polyps within the rectum and distal part of the colon. A slender, hollow, lighted tube is placed into the rectum, allowing the physician to look for polyps or other abnormalities. The sigmoidoscope is shorter than the colonoscope.

Solar irradiation:
See UV radiation.

Solid fuels:
Solid materials burned usually for heating purposes, including wood, peat, charcoal, coal, and grains. In certain conditions, excess exposure can be an important risk factor for lung cancer.

Survival (rate, estimate):
The proportion (or percentage) of persons with a given cancer who are still alive after a specified time period (e.g., 1, 3, or 5 years) following a diagnosis.

Targeted therapy:
A cancer treatment that uses drugs or other substances to identify and attack cancer cells while avoiding harm to normal cells better than many other cancer treatments. Some targeted therapies block the mechanisms involved in the growth and spread of cancer cells. Other types of targeted therapies help the immune system kill cancer cells or deliver toxic substances directly to cancer cells.

Ultraviolet (UV) radiation:
Invisible rays that are part of the energy that comes from the sun. UV radiation also comes from sun lamps and tanning beds. UV radiation can damage the skin, lead to premature aging, and cause melanoma and other types of skin cancer.

Vital registration:
The continuous, permanent, compulsory and universal recording of the occurrence and characteristics of vital events (e.g. births and deaths) pertaining to the population, as provided through decree or regulation in accordance with the legal requirements of a country.

Wilms tumor:
A type of kidney cancer that usually occurs in children younger than 5 years of age.

Years of life lost (YLL):
A statistic that measures the burden of premature death in a population due to a specific cause (such as cancer) within a specified time frame by aggregating the difference between expected life span and years lived among those who died due to the cause of interest.

Please refer to the **U.S. National Cancer Institute's "Dictionary of Cancer Terms"** for additional definitions (http://www.cancer.gov/dictionary).

SOURCES AND METHODS

A note about maps in this edition of *The Cancer Atlas:* Many maps throughout the *Atlas* were created using data from GLOBOCAN, a database of estimated cancer statistics created and maintained by the International Agency for Research on Cancer. A full description of the methods for creating these estimates can be found on the GLOBOCAN website (*http://globocan.iarc.fr/ Pages/DataSource_and_methods.aspx*).

Introduction

Photo:
Candlelight image courtesy of Global Relay For Life, American Cancer Society, 2014.

RISK FACTORS

Section Divider:
Ng M, Fleming T, Robinson M, et al. Global, regional, and national prevalence of overweight and obesity in children and adults during 1980-2013: a systematic analysis for the Global Burden of Disease Study 2013. *Lancet.* 2014 May 28. [Epub ahead of print].

Chan M. *Obesity: Trouble is on the way.* Lecture delivered to the Women's International Forum. New York. September 21, 2012. Available from: *http://www.who.int/dg/speeches/2012/ forum_20120921/en/*, accessed on June 17, 2014.

Overview of Risk Factors

Percent of cancer deaths due to smoking:
Ezzati M, Henley SJ, Lopez AD, Thun MJ. Role of smoking in global and regional cancer epidemiology: current patterns and data needs. *Int J Cancer.* 2005;116(6):963-71.

Text:
Haenszel W, Kurihara M. Studies of Japanese migrants. I. Mortality from cancer and other diseases among Japanese in the United States. *J Natl Cancer Inst.* 1968;40(1):43-68.

International Agency for Research on Cancer. *World Cancer Report 2014.* Lyon: International Agency for Research on Cancer; 2014.

Cogliano VJ, Baan R, Straif K, et al. Preventable exposures associated with human cancers. *J Natl Cancer Inst.* 2011;103(24):1827-39.

Ezzati M, Henley SJ, Lopez AD, Thun MJ. Role of smoking in global and regional cancer epidemiology: current patterns and data needs. *Int J Cancer.* 2005;116(6):963-71.

Thun MJ, Jemal A. How much of the decrease in cancer death rates in the United States is attributable to reductions in tobacco smoking? *Tob Control.* 2006;15(5):345-7.

Rushton L, Hutchings SJ, Fortunato L, et al. Occupational cancer burden in Great Britain. *Br J Cancer.* 2012;107 Suppl 1:S3-7.

Park J, Hisanaga N, Kim Y. Transfer of occupational health problems from a developed to a developing country: lessons from the Japan-South Korea experience. *Am J Ind Med.* 2009;52(8):625-32.

de Martel C, Ferlay J, Franceschi S, et al. Global burden of cancers attributable to infections in 2008: a review and synthetic analysis. *Lancet Oncol.* 2012;13(6):607-15.

Vineis P, Xun W. The emerging epidemic of environmental cancers in developing countries. *Ann Oncol.* 2009;20(2):205-12.

Figure 1:
Waterhouse J, Muir CS, Correa P, Powell J (Eds). *Cancer Incidence in Five Continents*, Vol. III. IARC Scientific Publications, No. 15. Lyon: IARC; 1976.

Figure 2:
Cogliano VJ, Baan R, Straif K, et al. Preventable exposures associated with human cancers. *J Natl Cancer Inst.* 2011;103(24):1827-39.

Ezzati M, Henley SJ, Lopez AD, Thun MJ. Role of smoking in global and regional cancer epidemiology: current patterns and data needs. *Int J Cancer.* 2005;116(6):963-71.

Vineis P, Alavanja M, Buffler P, et al. Tobacco and cancer: recent epidemiological evidence. *J Natl Cancer Inst.* 2004;96(2):99-106.

Figure 3:
Case RAM, Hosker ME, McDonald DB, Pearson JT. Tumours of the urinary bladder in workmen engaged in the manufacture and use of certain dyestuff intermediates in the British chemical industry. Part I. The role of aniline, benzidine, alpha-naphthylamine, and beta-naphthylamine. *Br J Ind Med.* 1954;11(2):75-104.

Figure 4:
Bruni L, Diaz M, Castellsagué X, et al. Cervical human papillomavirus prevalence in 5 continents: meta-analysis of 1 million women with normal cytological findings. *J Infect Dis.* 2010;202(12):1789-99.

Figure 5:
World Cancer Research Fund / American Institute for Cancer Research. *Food, Nutrition, Physical Activity, and the Prevention of Cancer: a Global Perspective.* Washington, DC: AICR; 2007.

Risks of Tobacco

Quote:
World Health Organization. *Statement by the Director-General to the Intergovernmental Negotiating Body on the WHO framework convention on tobacco control at its fifth session.* Available at: *http://apps.who.int/gb/fctc/PDF/inb5/ einb5d7.pdf.* Accessed July 11, 2014.

Deaths due to tobacco use in the 21st century:
Eriksen M, Mackay J, Ross H. *The Tobacco Atlas.* 4th edition. Atlanta: American Cancer Society; 2012.

Waterpipe use in young adults:
Akl EA, Gunukula SK, Aleem S, et al. The prevalence of waterpipe tobacco smoking among the general and specific populations: a systematic review. *BMC Public Health.* 2011;11:244.

Warren CW, Lea V, Lee J, et al. Change in tobacco use among 13-15 year olds between 1999 and 2008: findings from the Global Youth Tobacco Survey. *Glob Health Promot.* 2009;16(2 Suppl):38-90.

Text:
Eriksen M, Mackay J, Ross H. *The Tobacco Atlas.* 4th edition. Atlanta: American Cancer Society; 2012.

Thun MJ, Carter BD, Feskanich D, et al. 50-year trends in smoking-related mortality in the United States. *N Engl J Med.* 2013;368(4):351-64.

International Agency for Research on Cancer. *IARC Monographs on the Evaluation of Carcinogenic Risks to Humans: Smokeless tobacco and some tobacco-specific N-nitrosamines.* Vol. 89. Lyon: IARC; 2007.

International Agency for Research on Cancer. *IARC Monographs on the Evaluation of Carcinogenic Risks to Humans: Tobacco smoke and involuntary smoking.* Vol. 83. Lyon: IARC; 2004.

Oberg M, Jaakkola MS, Woodward A, et al. Worldwide burden of disease from exposure to second-hand smoke: a retrospective analysis of data from 192 countries. *Lancet.* 2011;377(9760):139-46.

SOURCES AND METHODS

Main Maps: Male and female (>15 years) smoking prevalence, 2013
Data were provided by the Institute for Health Metrics and Evaluation, 2014.

Figure 1:
Global Burden of Disease Study 2010. *Global Burden of Disease Study 2010 (GBD 2010) Results by Risk Factor 1990-2010.* Seattle: Institute for Health Metrics and Evaluation (IHME); 2012.

Figure 2:
Giovino GA, Mirza SA, Samet JM, et al. Tobacco use in 3 billion individuals from 16 countries: an analysis of nationally representative cross-sectional household surveys. *Lancet.* 2012; 380(9842):668-79.

Figure 3:
Warren CW, Lea V, Lee J, et al. Change in tobacco use among 13-15 year olds between 1999 and 2008: findings from the Global Youth Tobacco Survey. *Glob Health Promot.* 2009; 16(2 Suppl):38-90.

Infection

Helicobacter pylori responsible for 90% of stomach cancers:
de Martel C, Forman D, Plummer M. Gastric cancer: epidemiology and risk factors. *Gastroenterol Clin North Am.* 2013;42(2):219-40.

Text:
de Martel C, Ferlay J, Franceschi S, et al. Global burden of cancers attributable to infections in 2008: a review and synthetic analysis. *Lancet Oncol.* 2012;13(6):607-15.

de Martel C, Forman D, Plummer M. Gastric cancer: epidemiology and risk factors. *Gastroenterol Clin North Am.* 2013;42(2):219-40.

Forman D, de Martel C, Lacey CJ, et al. Global burden of human papillomavirus and related diseases. *Vaccine.* 2012;30 Suppl 5:F12-23.

International Agency for Research on Cancer. *IARC Monographs on the Evaluation of Carcinogenic Risks to Humans: Biological agents.* Vol. 100B. Lyon: IARC; 2012.

Map:
de Martel C, Ferlay J, Franceschi S, et al. Global burden of cancers attributable to infections in 2008: a review and synthetic analysis. *Lancet Oncol.* 2012;13(6):607-15.

Figure 1:
de Martel C, Ferlay J, Franceschi S, et al. Global burden of cancers attributable to infections in 2008: a review and synthetic analysis. *Lancet Oncol.* 2012;13(6):607-15.

Diet, Body Mass, and Physical Activity

Quote:
Hippocrates. *Hippocratic Writings.* Chicago: Encyclopedia Britannica; 1955.

In some countries 60% of adults are overweight or obese:
World Health Organization. *Global Health Observatory Data Repository, Overweight (Body Mass Index > 25) Data by Country, 2008* [online database]. Available from: *http://apps. who.int/ghodata/*, accessed November 9, 2012.

Text:
Baan R, Straif K, Grosse Y, et al. Carcinogenicity of alcoholic beverages. *Lancet Oncol.* 2007;8(4): 292-3.

Boffetta P, Hashibe M, La Vecchia C, et al. The burden of cancer attributable to alcohol drinking. *Int J Cancer.* 2006;119(4): 884-7.

Esposito K, Chiodini P, Colao A, Lenzi A, Giugliano D. Metabolic syndrome and risk of cancer: a systematic review and meta-analysis. *Diabetes Care.* 2012;35(11): 2402-11.

Esposito K, Ciardiello F, Giugliano D. Unhealthy diets: a common soil for the association of metabolic syndrome and cancer. *Endocrine.* Epub 2014 Jan 10.

International Agency for Research on Cancer. *IARC Monographs on the Evaluation of Carcinogenic Risks to Humans: Personal Habits and Indoor Combustions.* Vol. 100E. Lyon, France: IARC; 2012.

Kushi LH, Doyle C, McCullough M, et al. American Cancer Society Guidelines on nutrition and physical activity for cancer prevention: reducing the risk of cancer with healthy food choices and physical activity. *CA Cancer J Clin.* 2012;62(1):30-67.

Rock CL, Doyle C, Demark-Wahnefried W, et al. Nutrition and physical activity guidelines for cancer survivors. *CA Cancer J Clin.* 2012;62(4): 243-74.

World Cancer Research Fund / American Institute for Cancer Research. *Food, Nutrition, Physical Activity, and the Prevention of Cancer: a Global Perspective.* Washington, DC: AICR; 2007.

World Health Organization. *Global Recommendations on Physical Activity for Health.* Geneva: World Health Organization; 2010.

World Health Organization. *Global Status Report on Noncommunicable Diseases.* Geneva: World Health Organization; 2010.

Maps:
World Health Organization. *Global Health Observatory Data Repository, Overweight (Body Mass Index > 25) Data by Country, 2008* [online database]. Available from: *http://apps. who.int/ghodata/*, accessed November 9, 2012.

Figure 1:
International Agency for Research on Cancer. *IARC Monographs on the Evaluation of Carcinogenic Risks to Humans: Personal Habits and Indoor Combustions.* Vol. 100E. Lyon: IARC; 2012.

World Cancer Research Fund/American Institute for Cancer Research. *Continuous Update Project Summary. Food, Nutrition, Physical Activity, and the Prevention of Pancreatic Cancer.* Washington, DC: AICR; 2012.

World Cancer Research Fund/American Institute for Cancer Research. *Continuous Update Project Report Summary. Food, Nutrition, Physical Activity, and the Prevention of Colorectal Cancer.* Washington, DC: AICR; 2011.

World Cancer Research Fund/American Institute for Cancer Research. *Continuous Update Project Report Summary. Food, Nutrition, Physical Activity, and the Prevention of Breast Cancer.* Washington, DC: AICR; 2010.

World Cancer Research Fund/American Institute for Cancer Research. *Food, Nutrition, Physical Activity, and the Prevention of Cancer: a Global Perspective.* Washington, DC: AICR; 2007.

Figure 2:
Renehan AG, Soerjomataram I, Tyson M, et al. Incident cancer burden attributable to excess body mass index in 30 European countries. *Int J Cancer.* 2010; 126(3):692-702.

World Cancer Research Fund / American Institute for Cancer Research. *Policy and action for cancer prevention. Food, nutrition, and physical activity: a Global Perspective.* Washington, DC: AICR; 2009.

Figure 3:
Lee IM, Shiroma EJ, Lobelo F, et al. Effect of physical inactivity on major non-communicable diseases worldwide: an analysis of burden of disease and life expectancy. *Lancet.* 2012;380(9838):219-29.

Ultraviolet Radiation

Quote:
Jorgensen CM. Scientific recommendations and human behaviour: sitting out in the sun. *Lancet.* 2002;360(9330):351-2.

Childhood sunburns increase skin cancer risk:
Green AC, Wallingford SC, McBride P. Childhood exposure to ultraviolet radiation and harmful skin effects: epidemiological evidence. *Prog Biophys Mol Biol.* 2011;107(3):349-55.

Text:
American Cancer Society. *Skin Cancer: Basal and Squamous Cell.* Available from: *http://www.cancer.org/Cancer/SkinCancer -BasalandSquamousCell/DetailedGuide/skin-cancer-basal-and -squamous-cell-what-is-basal-and-squamous-cell*, accessed October 4, 2012.

Baade PD, Green AC, Smithers BM, Aitken JF. Trends in melanoma incidence among children: possible influence of sun-protection programs. *Expert Rev Anticancer Ther.* 2011;11(5):661-4.

Douglass A, Fioletov V, Godin-Beekmann S, et al. Stratospheric ozone and surface ultraviolet radiation. In: *Scientific Assessment of Ozone Depletion, Global Ozone Research and Monitoring Project-Report No. 52.* Geneva: World Meteorological Organization; 2010.

Ferlay J, Soerjomataram I, Ervik M, et al. GLOBOCAN 2012 v1.0, Cancer Incidence and Mortality Worldwide: IARC CancerBase No. 11 [Internet]. Available from: *http://globocan. iarc.fr*, accessed December 12, 2013.

Gallagher RP, Rivers JK, Lee TK, et al. Broad-spectrum sunscreen use and the development of new nevi in white children: A randomized controlled trial. *JAMA.* 2000;283(22):2955-60.

Green AC, Wallingford SC, McBride P. Childhood exposure to ultraviolet radiation and harmful skin effects: epidemiological evidence. *Prog Biophys Mol Biol.* 2011;107(3):349-55.

Green AC, Williams GM, Logan V, Strutton GM. Reduced melanoma after regular sunscreen use: randomized trial follow-up. *J Clin Oncol.* 2011;29(3):257-63.

International Agency for Research on Cancer. *IARC Monographs on the Evaluation of Carcinogenic Risks to Humans: Solar and Ultraviolet Radiation.* Vol. 100D. Lyon, France: IARC; 2012.

Lucas R, McMichael T, Smith W, Armstrong B. *Solar Ultraviolet Radiation: Global Burden of Disease from solar ultraviolet radiation. Environmental Burden of Disease Series, No. 13.* Geneva: World Health Organization; 2006.

The International Agency for Research on Cancer Working Group on Artificial Ultraviolet (UV) Light and Skin Cancer. The association of use of sunbeds with cutaneous malignant melanoma and other skin cancers: A systematic review. *Int J Cancer.* 2007;120(5):1116-22.

Whiteman DC, Whiteman CA, Green AC. Childhood sun exposure as a risk factor for melanoma: A systematic review of epidemiologic studies. *Cancer Causes Control.* 2001;12(1):69-82.

Map:
Ferlay J, Soerjomataram I, Ervik M, et al. GLOBOCAN 2012 v1.0, Cancer Incidence and Mortality Worldwide: IARC CancerBase No. 11 [Internet]. Available from: *http://globocan. iarc.fr*, accessed December 12, 2013.

Figure 1:
Bentzen J, Kjellberg J, Thorgaard C, et al. Costs of illness for melanoma and nonmelanoma skin cancer in Denmark. *Eur J Cancer Prev.* 2013;22(6):569-76.

Bickers DR, Lim HW, Margolis D, et al. The burden of skin diseases: 2004 a joint project of the American Academy of Dermatology Association and the Society for Investigative Dermatology. *J Am Acad Dermatol.* 2006;55(3):490-500.

Fransen M, Karahalios A, Sharma N, et al. Non-melanoma skin cancer in Australia. *Med J Aust.* 2012;197(10):565-8.

Souza RJ, Mattedi AP, Correa MP, et al. An estimate of the cost of treating non-melanoma skin cancer in the state of Sao Paulo, Brazil. *An Bras Dermatol.* 2011;86(4):657-662.

Tinghog G, Carlsson P, Synnerstad I, Rosdahl I. Societal cost of skin cancer in Sweden in 2005. *Acta Derm Venereol.* 2008;88(5):467-73.

Figure 2:
Boldeman C, Jansson B, Dal H, Ullen H. Sunbed use among Swedish adolescents in the 1990s: A decline with an unchanged relationship to health risk behaviors. *Scand J Public Health.* 2003;31(3):233-7.

Guy GP Jr, Tai E, Richardson LC. Use of indoor tanning devices by high school students in the United States, 2009. *Prev Chronic Dis.* 2011;8(5):A116.

Koster B, Thorgaard C, Clemmensen IH, Philip A. Sunbed use in the Danish population in 2007: A cross-sectional study. *Prev Med.* 2009;48(3):288-90.

Ontario Sun Safety Working Group. *National Sun Survey Highlights Report 2008.* 2008. Available from: http://www.uvnetwork.ca/ NationalSunSurveyHighlightsReport20080710.pdf, accessed October 9, 2012.

Figure 3:
Ferlay J, Bray F, Steliarova-Foucher E, Forman D. Cancer Incidence in Five Continents, CI5*plus:* IARC CancerBase [Internet]. Lyon, France: International Agency for Research on Cancer; 2014. Available from: http://ci5.iarc.fr, accessed December 12, 2013.

Reproductive and Hormonal Factors
Quote:
Collaborative Group on Hormonal Factors in Breast Cancer. Breast cancer and breastfeeding: Collaborative reanalysis of individual data from 47 epidemiological studies in 30 countries, including 50302 women with breast cancer and 96973 women without the disease. *Lancet.* 2002; 360(9328):187-95.

Fertility rates have declined by 50% in some countries:
United Nations Department of Economic and Social Affairs Population Division. *World Fertility Patterns 2009.* 2010. Available from: *http://www.un.org/esa/population/publications/ worldfertility2009/worldfertility2009.htm,* accessed August 15, 2014.

Text:
Ma H, Bernstein L, Pike MC, et al. Age at first birth, parity and risk of breast cancer: A meta-analysis of 8 studies from the Nordic countries. *Int J Cancer.* 1990; 46(4):597-603.

Collaborative Group on Hormonal Factors in Breast Cancer. Breast cancer and breastfeeding: Collaborative reanalysis of individual data from 47 epidemiological studies in 30 countries, including 50 302 women with breast cancer and 96 973 women without the disease. *Lancet.* 2002; 360(9328):187-95.

Pike MC, Wu AH, Spicer DV, et al. Estrogens, progestins, and risk of breast cancer. In: *Ernst Shering Foundation Symposium Proceedings,* Vol. 1. Berlin: Springer Verlag; 2007; pp. 127-50.

Collaborative Group on Hormonal Factors in Breast Cancer. Breast cancer and hormonal contraceptives: Collaborative reanalysis of individual data on 53 297 women with breast cancer and 100 239 women without breast cancer from 54 epidemiological studies. *Lancet.* 1996; 347:1713-27.

Beral V. Breast cancer and hormone-replacement therapy in the Million Women Study. *Lancet.* 2003; 362(9382):419-27.

Grosse Y, Baan R, Straif K, et al. A review of human carcinogens—Part A: Pharmaceuticals. *Lancet Oncol.* 2009;10(1):13-4.

Maps:
United Nations Department of Economic and Social Affairs Population Division. *World Fertility Patterns 2009.* 2010. Available from: *http://www.un.org/esa/population/publications/ worldfertility2009/worldfertility2009.htm,* accessed August 15, 2012.

Figure 1:
Tanner JM. Trend towards earlier menarche in London, Oslo, Copenhagen, the Netherlands and Hungary. *Nature.* 1973; 243:95-6.

Zacharias L, Wurtman RJ. Age at menarche: Genetic and environmental influences. *N Engl J Med.* 1969; 280:868-75.

Figure 2:
Collaborative Group on Hormonal Factors in Breast Cancer. Breast cancer and hormonal contraceptives: collaborative reanalysis of individual data on 53 297 women with breast cancer and 100 239 women without breast cancer from 54 epidemiological studies. *Lancet.* 1996; 347:1713-27.

Collaborative Group on Hormonal Factors in Breast Cancer. Breast cancer and hormone replacement therapy: collaborative reanalysis of data from 51 epidemiological studies of 52 705 women with breast cancer and 108 411 women without breast cancer. *Lancet.* 1997;350(9084):1047-59.

Collaborative Group on Hormonal Factors in Breast Cancer. Breast cancer and breastfeeding: Collaborative reanalysis of individual data from 47 epidemiological studies in 30 countries, including 50 302 women with breast cancer and 96 973 women without the disease. *Lancet.* 2002; 360(9328):187-95.

Ewertz M, Duffy SW, Adami HO, et al. Age at first birth, parity and risk of breast cancer: a meta-analysis of 8 studies from the Nordic countries. *Int J Cancer.* 1990; 46(4):597-603.

Environmental and Occupational Pollutants
Quote:
International Agency for Research on Cancer. *Press Release: Outdoor air pollution a leading environmental cause of cancer deaths.* 2013. Available from: *http://www.iarc.fr/en/ media-centre/iarcnews/pdf/pr221_E.pdf,* accessed August 18, 2014.

Text:
Benbrahim-Tallaa L, Baan RA, Grosse Y, et al. Carcinogenicity of diesel-engine and gasoline-engine exhausts and some nitroarenes. *Lancet Oncol.* 2012;13: 663-4.

Cantor KP, Lubin JH. Arsenic, internal cancers, and issues in inference from studies of low-level exposures in human populations. *Toxicol Appl Pharmacol.* 2007;222: 252-7.

Darby S, Hill D, Deo H, et al. Residential radon and lung cancer: Detailed results of a collaborative analysis of individual data on 7148 persons with lung cancer and 14,208 persons without lung cancer from 13 epidemiologic studies in Europe. *Scand J Work Environ Health.* 2006; 32(Suppl 1):1-83.

Field RW, Steck DJ, Smith BJ, et al. Residential radon gas exposure and lung cancer: The Iowa Radon Lung Cancer Study. *Am J Epidemiol.* 2000;151(11):1091-102. International Agency for Research on Cancer. *IARC monographs on the evaluation of the carcinogenic risk of chemicals to humans: Indoor air pollution from heating and cooking: some solid fuels and cooking oil fumes.* Vol. 95. Lyon, France: IARC; 2006.

Loomis D, Grosse Y, Lauby-Secretan B, et al. The carcinogenicity of outdoor air pollution. *Lancet Oncol.* 2013; 14: 1262-3.

Santana VS, Ribiero FSN. Occupational cancer burden in developing countries and the problem of informal workers. *Environmental Health.* 2011; 10(Suppl 1):S10.

Map: Mean annual PM2.5 levels
World Health Organization. *Global Health Observatory Data Repository, Ambient air pollution database, May 2014* [online database]. Available from: *http://apps.who.int/gho/data/ node.main.152?lang=en,* accessed July 9, 2014.

Figure 1:
(Heading) World Health Organization. *Household Air Pollution and Health.* Available from: *http://www.who.int/mediacentre/ factsheets/fs292/en/,* accessed August 19, 2014.

World Health Organization. *Global Health Observatory Data Repository, Population using solid fuels (estimates), 2010, data by country* [online database]. Available from: *http://apps.who.int/gho/data/view.main.1701?lang=en,* accessed July 9, 2014.

Figure 2:
Boffetta P, Kogevinas M, Saracci R, et al. Occupational carcinogens. In: *Encyclopedia of occupational health and safety.* Vol. 2, Cancer. Stellman JM (Ed). Geneva, Switzerland: International Labor Organization; 2011.

Figure 3:
Park EK, Takahashi K, Hoshuyama T, et al. Global magnitude of reported and unreported mesothelioma. *Environ Health Perspect.* 2011;119:514-8.

Figure 4:
Virta RL. *Worldwide asbestos supply and consumption trends from 1900 through 2003: U.S. Geological Survey Circular 1298.* Reston, VA; United States Geological Survey; 2006. Available from: *http://pubs.usgs.gov/circ/2006/1298/ c1298.pdf,* accessed July 25, 2014.

Human Carcinogens Identified by the IARC Monographs Program
Over 100 carcinogenic agents:
Cogliano VJ, Baan R, Straif K, et al. Preventable exposures associated with human cancers. *J Natl. Cancer Inst.* 2011;103:1827-39.

Text:
International Agency for Research on Cancer. *IARC monographs for the evaluation of carcinogenic risks to humans.* Available from: *http://monographs.iarc.fr/,* accessed July 25, 2014.

Figure:
Cogliano VJ, Baan R, Straif K, et al. Preventable exposures associated with human cancers. *J Natl. Cancer Inst.* 2011;103:1827-39.

THE BURDEN
Section Divider
Stewart BW, Wild CP (Eds). *World Cancer Report 2014.* Lyon: IARC; 2014.

Bray F, Jemal A, Grey N, et al. Global cancer transitions according to the Human Development Index (2008-2030): a population-based study. *Lancet Oncol.* 2012; 13(8): 790-801.

The Burden of Cancer

Cancer the most important cause of death worldwide:
World Health Organization. *Disease and injury regional estimates, 2000–2011. Global Summary Statistics.* Available from: http://www.who.int/healthinfo/global_burden _disease/estimates_regional_2000_2011/en/, accessed July 25, 2014.

Quote:
World Health Organization. *Message of the WHO Regional Director, Dr Luis Gomes Sambo, on the occasion of World Cancer Day 2014.* 2014. Available from: http://www.afro .who.int/en/rdo/speeches/3980-world-cancer-day-2014.html, accessed August 15, 2014.

Text:
Ferlay J, Soerjomataram I, Ervik M, et al. GLOBOCAN 2012 v1.0, Cancer Incidence and Mortality Worldwide: IARC CancerBase No. 11 [Internet]. Lyon: IARC; 2013. Available from: http://globocan.iarc.fr, accessed May 19, 2014.

Map: Years of life lost due to cancer
Ferlay J, Shin HR, Bray F, et al. GLOBOCAN 2008 v1.2: Cancer incidence and mortality worldwide: IARC CancerBase No. 10. Lyon: IARC; 2010.

Map: Most commonly diagnosed cancers
Ferlay J, Soerjomataram I, Ervik M, et al. GLOBOCAN 2012 v1.0, Cancer Incidence and Mortality Worldwide: IARC CancerBase No. 11 [Internet]. Lyon: IARC; 2013. Available from: http://globocan.iarc.fr, accessed May 19, 2014.

Figures 1 and 2:
Ferlay J, Soerjomataram I, Ervik M, et al. GLOBOCAN 2012 v1.0, Cancer Incidence and Mortality Worldwide: IARC CancerBase No. 11 [Internet]. Lyon: IARC; 2013. Available from: http://globocan.iarc.fr, accessed May 19, 2014.

Figure 3:
World Health Organization. *Disease and injury regional estimates, 2000–2011. Global summary statistics.* Available from: http://www.who.int/healthinfo/global_burden _disease/estimates_regional_2000_2011/en/, accessed July 25, 2014.

Lung Cancer

One-third of new lung cancer cases worldwide occur in China
Ferlay J, Soerjomataram I, Ervik M, et al. GLOBOCAN 2012 v1.0, Cancer Incidence and Mortality Worldwide: IARC CancerBase No. 11 [Internet]. Lyon: IARC; 2013. Available from: http://globocan.iarc.fr, accessed May 19, 2014.

Text:
Ferlay J, Soerjomataram I, Ervik M, et al. GLOBOCAN 2012 v1.0, Cancer Incidence and Mortality Worldwide: IARC CancerBase No. 11 [Internet]. Lyon: IARC; 2013. Available from: http://globocan.iarc.fr, accessed May 19, 2014.

Ferlay J, Bray F, Steliarova-Foucher E, Forman D. Cancer Incidence in Five Continents, CI5plus: IARC CancerBase [Internet]. Lyon, France: International Agency for Research on Cancer; 2014. Available from: http://ci5.iarc.fr, accessed May 23, 2014.

Maps:
Ferlay J, Soerjomataram I, Ervik M, et al. GLOBOCAN 2012 v1.0, Cancer Incidence and Mortality Worldwide: IARC CancerBase No. 11 [Internet]. Lyon: IARC; 2013. Available from: http://globocan.iarc.fr, accessed May 19, 2014.

Figures 1 and 3:
Ferlay J, Soerjomataram I, Ervik M, et al. GLOBOCAN 2012 v1.0, Cancer Incidence and Mortality Worldwide: IARC CancerBase No. 11 [Internet]. Lyon: IARC; 2013. Available from: http://globocan.iarc.fr, accessed May 19, 2014.

Figure 2:
Ferlay J, Bray F, Steliarova-Foucher E, Forman D. Cancer Incidence in Five Continents, CI5plus: IARC CancerBase [Internet]. Lyon, France: International Agency for Research on Cancer; 2014. Available from: http://ci5.iarc.fr, accessed May 23, 2014.

Breast Cancer

Quote:
Schultz, DW. *Every Woman Should Know.* Available from: http://wassermanschultz.house.gov/2010/03/susan-g-komen -for-the-cure-every-woman-should-know.shtml, accessed June 10, 2014.

New breast cancer cases and deaths:
Ferlay J, Soerjomataram I, Ervik M, et al. GLOBOCAN 2012 v1.0, Cancer Incidence and Mortality Worldwide: IARC CancerBase No. 11 [Internet]. Lyon: IARC; 2013. Available from: http://globocan.iarc.fr, accessed May 19, 2014.

Text:
Ferlay J, Bray F, Steliarova-Foucher E, Forman D. *Cancer Incidence in Five Continents*, CI5plus: IARC CancerBase [Internet]. Lyon, France: International Agency for Research on Cancer; 2014. Available from: http://ci5.iarc.fr, accessed May 23, 2014.

Ferlay J, Soerjomataram I, Ervik M, et al. GLOBOCAN 2012 v1.0, Cancer Incidence and Mortality Worldwide: IARC CancerBase No. 11 [Internet]. Lyon: IARC; 2013. Available from: http://globocan.iarc.fr, accessed May 19, 2014.

Maps and Figures 1 and 3:
Ferlay J, Soerjomataram I, Ervik M, et al. GLOBOCAN 2012 v1.0, Cancer Incidence and Mortality Worldwide: IARC CancerBase No. 11 [Internet]. Lyon: IARC; 2013. Available from: http://globocan.iarc.fr, accessed May 19, 2014.

Figure 2:
Ferlay J, Bray F, Steliarova-Foucher E, Forman D. *Cancer Incidence in Five Continents*, CI5plus: IARC CancerBase [Internet]. Lyon, France: International Agency for Research on Cancer; 2014. Available from: http://ci5.iarc.fr, accessed May 23, 2014.

World Health Organization. *WHO Cancer Mortality Database* [internet]. Available from: http://www-dep.iarc.fr/WHOdb/ WHOdb.htm, accessed May 27, 2014.

Cancer in Children

Quote:
Albert Einstein Quotes. Available from: https://www.goodreads .com/quotes/624713-there-is-no-great-discoveries-and -advances-as-long-as, accessed May 14, 2014.

Over half of childhood cancers are leukemias, lymphomas, or brain tumors:
Parkin DM, Kramárová E, Draper GJ, et al (Eds). *International Incidence of Childhood Cancer*. Vol. 2 (IARC Scientific Publications No. 144). Lyon: IARC; 1998.

Text:
Baade PD, Youlden DR, Valery PC, et al. Trends in incidence of childhood cancer in Australia, 1983-2006. *Br J Cancer.* 2010;102(3):620-6.

Bao PP, Zheng Y, Wang CF, et al. Time trends and characteristics of childhood cancer among children age 0-14 in Shanghai. *Pediatr Blood Cancer.* 2009;53:13-16.

Bunin GR. Nongenetic causes of childhood cancers: evidence from international variation, time trends, and risk factor studies. *Toxicol Appl Pharmacol.* 2004;199(2):91-103.

de Moor JS, Mariotto AB, Parry C, et al. Cancer survivors in the United States: Prevalence across the survivorship trajectory and implications for care. *Cancer Epidemiol Biomarkers Prev.* 2013;22:561-70.

Ferlay J, Soerjomataram I, Ervik M, et al. GLOBOCAN 2012 v1.0, Cancer Incidence and Mortality Worldwide: IARC CancerBase No. 11 [Internet]. Lyon, France: International Agency for Research on Cancer; 2013. Available from: http://globocan.iarc.fr, accessed December 20, 2013.

Forman D, Bray F, Brewster DH, et al (Eds). *Cancer Incidence in Five Continents*, Vol. X. Lyon: IARC, 2013. Available from: http://ci5.iarc.fr, accessed December 6, 2013.

Kaatsch P, Steliarova-Foucher E, Crocetti E, et al. Time trends of cancer incidence in European children (1978-1997): report from the Automated Childhood Cancer Information System project. *Eur J Cancer.* 2006;42(13):1961-71.

Kohler BA, Ward E, McCarthy BJ, et al. Annual report to the nation on the status of cancer, 1975-2007, featuring tumors of the brain and other nervous system. *J Natl Cancer Inst.* 2011;103:714-36.

Magrath I, Steliarova-Foucher E, Epelman S, et al. Paediatric cancer in low-income and middle-income countries. *Lancet Oncol.* 2013;14(3):e104-16.

Oeffinger KC, Mertens AC, Sklar CA, et al. Chronic health conditions in adult survivors of childhood cancer. *N Engl J Med.* 2006;355:1572-82.

Parkin DM, Kramárová E, Draper GJ, et al (Eds). *International Incidence of Childhood Cancer*. Vol. 2 (IARC Scientific Publications No. 144). Lyon: IARC; 1998.

Stiller CA. Epidemiology and genetics of childhood cancer. *Oncogene.* 2004; 23:6429-44.

Stiller CA, Desandes E, Danon SE, et al. Cancer incidence and survival in European adolescents (1978-1997): Report from the Automated Childhood Cancer Information System project. *Eur J Cancer.* 2006;42:2006-18.

Stiller CA, Kroll ME, Eatock EM. Survival from childhood cancer. In: *Childhood Cancer in Britain: Incidence, survival, mortality.* Stiller CA (Editor). Oxford: Oxford UP; 2007. pp 131-204.

Vassal G, Zwaan CM, Ashley D, et al. Improving cancer care for children and young people: New drugs for children and adolescents with cancer: the need for novel development pathways. *Lancet Oncol.* 2013; 14: e117-24.

Wakeford R. The risk of childhood leukaemia following exposure to ionising radiation--a review. *J Radiol Prot.* 2013;33(1):1-25.

Figure 1:
Ferlay J, Soerjomataram I, Ervik M, et al. GLOBOCAN 2012 v1.0, Cancer Incidence and Mortality Worldwide: IARC CancerBase No. 11 [Internet]. Lyon: International Agency for Research on Cancer; 2013. Available from: http://globocan. iarc.fr, accessed December 20, 2013.

Figure 2:
Baade PD, Youlden DR, Valery PC, et al. Trends in incidence of childhood cancer in Australia, 1983-2006. *Br J Cancer.* 2010;102(3):620-6.

Bao PP, Zheng Y, Wang CF, et al. Time trends and characteristics of childhood cancer among children age 0-14 in Shanghai. *Pediatr Blood Cancer.* 2009;53:13-6.

Fajardo-Gutiérrez A, Juarez-Ocaña S, González-Miranda G, et al. Incidence of cancer in children residing in ten jurisdictions of the Mexican Republic: Importance of the Cancer registry (a population-based study). *BMC Cancer.* 2007; 7:68

Kohler BA, Ward E, McCarthy BJ, et al. Annual report to the nation on the status of cancer, 1975–2007, featuring tumors of the brain and other nervous system. *J Natl Cancer Inst.* 2011; 103:714-36.

Kaatsch P, Spix J. *German Childhood Cancer Registry - Annual Report 2011 (1980-2010).* Mainz: University Medical Center of the Johannes Gutenberg University; 2012. Available from *http://www.kinderkrebsregister.de/extern/ veroeffentlichungen/jahresberichte/aktueller-jahresbericht/index. html?L=1*, accessed May 30, 2013.

Lacour B, Guyot-Goubin A, Guissou S, et al. Incidence of childhood cancer in France: National Children Cancer Registries, 2000–2004. *Eur J Cancer Prev.* 2010;19(3):173-81.

Moradi A, Semnani S, Roshandel G, et al. Incidence of childhood cancers in Golestan province of Iran. *Iran J Pediatr.* 2010;20(3):335-342.

Moreno F, Loria D, Abriata G, et al. Childhood cancer: Incidence and early deaths in Argentina, 2000-2008. *Eur J Cancer.* 2013;49(2):465-73.

Parkin DM, Ferlay J, Hamdi-Chérif M, et al (Eds). Childhood cancer. In: *Cancer in Africa, epidemiology and prevention.* IARC Scientific Publications No. 153. Lyon: IARC; 2003. pp. 381-96.

Swaminathan R, Rama R, Shanta V. Childhood cancers in Chennai, India, 1990–2001: Incidence and survival. *Int J Cancer.* 2008;122(11):2607-11.

Wiangnon S, Veerakul G, Nuchprayoon I, et al. Childhood Cancer Incidence and Survival 2003-2005, Thailand: Study from the Thai Pediatric Oncology Group. *Asian Pac J Cancer Prev.* 2011;12(9):2215-20.

Figure 3:
Baade PD, Youlden DR, Valery PC, et al. Population-based survival estimates for childhood cancer in Australia during the period 1997–2006. *Br J Cancer.* 2010; 103(11):1663-70.

Bao PP, Zheng Y, Wu CX, et al. Population-based survival for childhood cancer patients diagnosed during 2002-2005 in Shanghai, China. Pediatr Blood Cancer. 2012;59(4):657-61.

Swaminathan R, Rama R, Shanta V. Childhood cancers in Chennai, India, 1990–2001: Incidence and survival. *Int J Cancer.* 2008;122(11):2607-11.

Wiangnon S, Veerakul G, Nuchprayoon I, et al. Childhood cancer incidence and survival 2003-2005, Thailand: Study from the Thai Pediatric Oncology Group. *Asian Pac J Cancer Prev.* 2011;12(9):2215-20.

Figure 4:
Ferlay J, Soerjomataram I, Ervik M, et al. GLOBOCAN 2012 v1.0, Cancer Incidence and Mortality Worldwide: IARC CancerBase No. 11 [Internet]. Lyon: International Agency for Research on Cancer; 2013. Available from: *http://globocan .iarc.fr*, accessed December 20, 2013.

Figure 5:
Fast Stats: An interactive tool for access to SEER cancer statistics. Surveillance Research Program, National Cancer Institute. Available from: *http://seer.cancer.gov/faststats*, accessed November 25, 2013.

Human Development Index Transitions

HDI transitions and cancer occurrence:
Bray F, Jemal A, Grey N, et al. Global cancer transitions according to the Human Development Index (2008-2030): a population-based study. *Lancet Oncol.* 2012;13(8):790-801.

Text:
Bray F, Jemal A, Grey N, et al. Global cancer transitions according to the Human Development Index (2008-2030): a population-based study. *Lancet Oncol.* 2012;13(8):790-801.

Ferlay J, Soerjomataram I, Ervik M, et al. GLOBOCAN 2012 v1.0, Cancer Incidence and Mortality Worldwide: IARC CancerBase No. 11 [Internet]. Available from: *http://globocan .iarc.fr*, accessed December 12, 2013.

Map:
United Nations Development Programme. *Human Development Report 2013.* New York: United Nations Development Programme; 2013. Available from: *http://hdr.undp.org/sites/default/files/reports/14/hdr2013_en _complete.pdf*, accessed May 14, 2014.

Figure 1:
Ferlay J, Soerjomataram I, Ervik M, et al. GLOBOCAN 2012 v1.0, Cancer Incidence and Mortality Worldwide: IARC CancerBase No. 11 [Internet]. Available from: *http://globocan .iarc.fr*, accessed May 14, 2014.

2025 projections provided by the International Agency for Research on Cancer, 2014.

Figure 2:
Ferlay J, Bray F, Steliarova-Foucher E, Forman D. Cancer Incidence in Five Continents, CI5plus: IARC CancerBase [Internet]. Lyon, France: International Agency for Research on Cancer; 2014. Available from: *http://ci5.iarc.fr*, accessed May 23, 2014.

Figure 3:
Ferlay J, Soerjomataram I, Ervik M, et al. GLOBOCAN 2012 v1.0, Cancer Incidence and Mortality Worldwide: IARC CancerBase No. 11 [Internet]. Available from: *http://globocan .iarc.fr*, accessed May 14, 2013.

Geographic Diversity: Overview

Quote:
Peto J. Cancer epidemiology in the last century and the next decade. *Nature.* 2001;411(6835):390-5.

Text:
de Martel C, Ferlay J, Franceschi S, et al. Global burden of cancers attributable to infections in 2008: a review and synthetic analysis. *Lancet Oncology.* 2012;13(6):607-15.

Danaei G, Vander Hoorn S, Lopez AD, et al. Causes of cancer in the world: comparative risk assessment of nine behavioural and environmental risk factors. *Lancet.* 2005;366(9499):1784-93.

Ferlay J, Soerjomataram I, Ervik M, et al. GLOBOCAN 2012 v1.0, Cancer Incidence and Mortality Worldwide: IARC CancerBase No. 11 [Internet]. Available from: *http://globocan .iarc.fr*, accessed March 20, 2013.

Peto J. Cancer epidemiology in the last century and the next decade. *Nature.* 2001;411(6835):390-5.

Maps:
Ferlay J, Soerjomataram I, Ervik M, et al. GLOBOCAN 2012 v1.0, Cancer Incidence and Mortality Worldwide: IARC CancerBase No. 11 [Internet]. Available from: *http://globocan .iarc.fr*, accessed March 20, 2013.

Figure 1:
Forman D, Bray F, Brewster DH, et al (Eds). Cancer Incidence in Five Continents, Vol. X (electronic version) Lyon, IARC; 2013. Available from: *http://ci5.iarc.fr*, accessed May 14, 2014.

Figure 2:
Danaei G, Vander Hoorn S, Lopez AD, et al. Causes of cancer in the world: comparative risk assessment of nine behavioural and environmental risk factors. *Lancet.* 2005;366(9499):1784-93.

de Martel C, Ferlay J, Franceschi S, et al. Global burden of cancers attributable to infections in 2008: a review and synthetic analysis. *Lancet Oncology.* 2012;13(6):607-15.

Geographic Diversity:
Cancer in Sub-Saharan Africa

Quote:
World Health Organization. *Preventing chronic diseases: A vital investment.* Geneva: World Health Organization; 2005. Available from: *http://www.who.int/chp/chronic_disease_report/ contents/foreword.pdf?ua=1*, accessed May 23, 2014.

Text:
de Martel C, Ferlay J, Franceschi S, et al. Global burden of cancers attributable to infections in 2008: A review and synthetic analysis. *Lancet Oncol.* 2013;13(6):607-615.

Ferlay J, Soerjomataram I, Ervik M, et al. GLOBOCAN 2012 v1.0, Cancer Incidence and Mortality Worldwide: IARC CancerBase No. 11 [Internet]. International Agency for Research on Cancer. *http://globocan.iarc.fr*, accessed December 12, 2013.

Maps and Figures 1 and 2:
Ferlay J, Soerjomataram I, Ervik M, et al. GLOBOCAN 2012 v1.0, Cancer Incidence and Mortality Worldwide: IARC CancerBase No. 11 [Internet]. International Agency for Research on Cancer. *http://globocan.iarc.fr*, accessed December 12, 2013.

Figure 3:
Chokunonga E, Borok M, Chirenje Z, et al. Trends in the incidence of cancer in the black population of Harare, Zimbabwe 1991-2010. *Int J Cancer.* 2013;133(7):721-9.

Geographic Diversity:
Cancer in Latin America and the Caribbean

Gallbladder rates in Chile
Ferlay J, Soerjomataram I, Ervik M, et al. GLOBOCAN 2012 v1.0, Cancer Incidence and Mortality Worldwide: IARC CancerBase No. 11 [Internet]. International Agency for Research on Cancer. *http://globocan.iarc.fr*, accessed December 12, 2013.

Text:
Ferlay J, Bray F, Steliarova-Foucher E, Forman D. Cancer Incidence in Five Continents, CI5plus: IARC CancerBase [Internet]. Lyon, France: International Agency for Research on Cancer; 2014. Available from: http://ci5.iarc.fr, accessed December 13, 2013.

Ferlay J, Soerjomataram I, Ervik M, et al. GLOBOCAN 2012 v1.0, Cancer Incidence and Mortality Worldwide: IARC CancerBase No. 11 [Internet]. International Agency for Research on Cancer. *http://globocan.iarc.fr*, accessed December 12, 2013.

International Agency for Research on Cancer. *Cancer Mortality Database.* Lyon; IARC; 2013 [internet]. Available from: *http://www-dep.iarc.fr/WHOdb/WHOdb.htm*, accessed December 13, 2013.

Map and Figure 1:
Ferlay J, Soerjomataram I, Ervik M, et al. GLOBOCAN 2012 v1.0, Cancer Incidence and Mortality Worldwide: IARC CancerBase No. 11 [Internet]. International Agency for Research on Cancer. *http://globocan.iarc.fr*, accessed December 12, 2013.

Figure 2:
Ferlay J, Bray F, Steliarova-Foucher E, Forman D. Cancer Incidence in Five Continents, CI5plus: IARC CancerBase [Internet]. Lyon, France: International Agency for Research on Cancer; 2014. Available from: *http://ci5.iarc.fr*, accessed December 13, 2013.

Figure 3:
International Agency for Research on Cancer. Cancer Mortality Database. Lyon; IARC; 2013 [internet]. Available from: *http://www-dep.iarc.fr/WHOdb/WHOdb.htm*, accessed December 13, 2013.

Geographic Diversity: Cancer in Northern America

Quote:
Broder S. Progress and Challenges in the National Cancer Program. In: *Origins of human cancer: a comprehensive review.* Brugge J, Curran T, Harlow E, McCormick F (Eds). Plainview, NY: Cold Spring Harbor Laboratory Press; 1991.

Lung cancer rates in Kentucky versus Utah:
Copeland G, Lake A, Firth R, et al (eds). *Cancer in North America: 2007-2011. Volume Two: Registry-specific cancer incidence in the United States and Canada.* Springfield, IL: North American Association of Central Cancer Registries; 2014.

Text:
Edwards BK, Noone AM, Mariotto AB, et al. Annual report to the nation on the status of cancer, 1975-2010, featuring prevalence of comorbidity and impact on survival among persons with lung, colorectal, breast, or prostate cancer. *Cancer.* 2013;120(9):1290–314.

Ferlay J, Soerjomataram I, Ervik M, et al. GLOBOCAN 2012 v1.0, Cancer Incidence and Mortality Worldwide: IARC CancerBase No. 11 [Internet]. International Agency for Research on Cancer. *http://globocan.iarc.fr*, accessed December 12, 2013.

Jemal A, Thun MJ, Ries LA, et al. Annual report to the nation on the status of cancer, 1975-2005, featuring trends in lung cancer, tobacco use, and tobacco control. *J Natl Cancer Inst.* 2008;100(23):1672-94.

Simard EP, Ward EM, Siegel R, Jemal A. Cancers with increasing incidence trends in the United States: 1999 through 2008. *CA Cancer J Clin.* 2012;62(2):118-28.

Ward E, Halpern M, Schrag N, et al. Association of insurance with cancer care utilization and outcomes. *CA Cancer J Clin.* 2008;58(1):9-31.

Map:
Copeland G, Lake A, Firth R, et al (eds). *Cancer in North America: 2007-2011. Volume Two: Registry-specific cancer incidence in the United States and Canada.* Springfield, IL: North American Association of Central Cancer Registries; 2014.

DATA QUALITY AND EXCLUSIONS:
Some states and provinces only met quality/fit-for-use standards for all years; years for which data did not meet quality standards are excluded. Arkansas rates are based on 2007–2009 data. Nevada rates are based on 2007-2010 data. Nunavut rates are based on 2007 data only. Minnesota, Quebec, and Puerto Rico were not included in *Cancer incidence in North America 2007-2011* data due to data issues.

Figure 1:
Ferlay J, Soerjomataram I, Ervik M, et al. GLOBOCAN 2012 v1.0, Cancer Incidence and Mortality Worldwide: IARC CancerBase No. 11 [Internet]. International Agency for Research on Cancer. *http://globocan.iarc.fr*, accessed December 12, 2013.

Figure 2:
Ferlay J, Bray F, Steliarova-Foucher E, Forman D. Cancer Incidence in Five Continents, CI5plus: IARC CancerBase [Internet]. Lyon, France: International Agency for Research on Cancer; 2014. Available from: *http://ci5.iarc.fr*, accessed December 13, 2013.

Figure 3:
Surveillance, Epidemiology, and End Results (SEER) Program (www.seer.cancer.gov) SEER*Stat Database: Mortality - All COD, Aggregated With State, Total U.S. (1969-2010) <Katrina/Rita Population Adjustment>, National Cancer Institute, DCCPS, Surveillance Research Program, Surveillance Systems Branch, released April 2013. Underlying mortality data provided by NCHS (www.cdc.gov/nchs).

Figure 4:
National Cancer Database, American College of Surgeons Commission on Cancer, 2011 Data Submission. American College of Surgeons, 2013.

METHODS:
Data included patients diagnosed in 2005 and 2006, and excluded patients within unknown stage, age, ZIP code, and race/ethnicity information. Patients who were of race/ethnicity other than white, black, or Hispanic were also excluded. Covariates included in the model included age, race, sex, ZIP code-based income and cancer site.

Geographic Diversity: Cancer in Southern, Eastern, and Southeastern Asia

Quote:
Hippocrates. Hippocratic writings. Lloyd GER (Ed). Harmondsworth, UK: Penguin; 1978.

Oral cancer in India:
Boffetta P, Hecht S, Gray N, et al. Smokeless tobacco and cancer. *Lancet Oncol.* 2008;9(7):667-75.

Text:
Boffetta P, Hecht S, Gray N, et al. Smokeless tobacco and cancer. *Lancet Oncol.* 2008;9(7):667-75.

Ferlay J, Soerjomataram I, Ervik M, et al. GLOBOCAN 2012 v1.0, Cancer Incidence and Mortality Worldwide: IARC CancerBase No. 11 [Internet]. International Agency for Research on Cancer. *http://globocan.iarc.fr*, accessed December 12, 2013.

Jemal A, Bray F, Center MM, et al. Global cancer statistics. *CA Cancer J Clin.* 2011;61(2):69-90.

Hwang EW, Cheung R. Global epidemiology of hepatitis B virus infection. *N A J Med Sci.* 2011;4(1):7-13.

Kimman M, Norman R, Jan S, et al. The burden of cancer in member countries of Southeast Asian Nations (ASEAN). *Asian Pac J Cancer Prev.* 2012;13: 411–20.

Sriplung H, Wiangnon S, Sontipong S, et al. Cancer incidence trends in Thailand, 1989-2000. *Asian Pac J Cancer Prev.*

WHO. Background document for including household air pollution as a regional target for prevention and control of non-communicable diseases. Part of Technical Working Group Meeting on Regional Action Plan and Targets for Prevention and Control of Non-communicable Diseases held at Bangkok,

Thailand from 11-13 June 2013. 2013. Available from *http://www.searo.who.int/entity/noncommunicable_diseases/events/ncd_twg_bangkok_technical_paper_household_air_pollution.pdf*, accessed May 14, 2014.

WHO. Resolution of the WHO Regional Committee on South East Asia: Regional action plan and targets for the control of non-communicable diseases- 2013-2030. SEA/R66/R6. 2013. Available from *http://www.searo.who.int/mediacentre/events/governance/rc/66/r6.pdf*, accessed May 14, 2014.

Maps and Figures 1 and 2:
Ferlay J, Soerjomataram I, Ervik M, et al. GLOBOCAN 2012 v1.0, Cancer Incidence and Mortality Worldwide: IARC CancerBase No. 11 [Internet]. International Agency for Research on Cancer. *http://globocan.iarc.fr*, accessed December 12, 2013.

Figure 3:
Ferlay J, Bray F, Steliarova-Foucher E, Forman D. Cancer Incidence in Five Continents, CI5plus: IARC CancerBase [Internet]. Lyon, France: International Agency for Research on Cancer; 2014. Available from: *http://ci5.iarc.fr*, accessed December 13, 2013.

Geographic Diversity: Cancer in Europe

Text:
Ferlay J, Soerjomataram I, Ervik M, et al. GLOBOCAN 2012 v1.0, Cancer Incidence and Mortality Worldwide: IARC CancerBase No. 11 [Internet]. International Agency for Research on Cancer. *http://globocan.iarc.fr*, accessed December 12, 2013.

Ferlay J, Steliarova-Foucher E, Lortet-Tieulent J, et al. Cancer incidence and mortality patterns in Europe: Estimates for 40 countries in 2012. *Eur J Cancer.* 2013 ;49(6):1374-403.

Lortet-Tieulent J, Renteria E, Sharp L, et al. Convergence of decreasing male and increasing female incidence rates in major tobacco-related cancers in Europe in 1988-2010. *Eur J Cancer.* 2013; pii: S0959-8049(13)00952-0.

Maps and Figures 1 and 2:
Ferlay J, Soerjomataram I, Ervik M, et al. GLOBOCAN 2012 v1.0, Cancer Incidence and Mortality Worldwide: IARC CancerBase No. 11 [Internet]. International Agency for Research on Cancer. *http://globocan.iarc.fr*, accessed December 12, 2013.

Figure 3:
International Agency for Research on Cancer. Cancer Mortality Database. Lyon; IARC; 2013 [internet]. Available from: *http://www-dep.iarc.fr/WHOdb/WHOdb.htm*, accessed December 13, 2013.

Figure 4:
Ferlay J, Bray F, Steliarova-Foucher E, Forman D. Cancer Incidence in Five Continents, CI5plus: IARC CancerBase [Internet]. Lyon, France: International Agency for Research on Cancer; 2014. Available from: *http://ci5.iarc.fr*, accessed December 13, 2013.

International Agency for Research on Cancer. Cancer Mortality Database. Lyon; IARC; 2013 [internet]. Available from: *http://www-dep.iarc.fr/WHOdb/WHOdb.htm*, accessed December 13, 2013.

Geographic Diversity: Cancer in Northern Africa, Central Asia, and West Asia

Quote:
Brown R, Kerr K, Haoudi A, Darzi A. Tackling cancer burden in the Middle East: Qatar as an example. *Lancet Oncol.* 2012;13(11):e501-8.

Esophageal cancer belt:

Ferlay J, Soerjomataram I, Ervik M, et al. GLOBOCAN 2012 v1.0, Cancer Incidence and Mortality Worldwide: IARC CancerBase No. 11 [Internet]. International Agency for Research on Cancer. http://globocan.iarc.fr, accessed April 4, 2014.

Eser S, Yakut C, Özdemir R, et al. Cancer incidence rates in Turkey in 2006: A detailed registry based estimation. *Asian Pac J Cancer Prev.* 2010;11(6):1731-9.

Text:

Boffetta P. Epidemiology of environmental and occupational cancer. *Oncogene.* 2004; 23:6392-403.

Boyle P, Levin B. *World Cancer Report 2008.* Lyon: IARC Press; 2008.

Center MM, Jemal A. International trends in liver cancer incidence rates. *Cancer Epidemiol Biomarkers Prev.* 2011;20:2362-8.

Ferlay J, Soerjomataram I, Ervik M, et al. GLOBOCAN 2012 v1.0, Cancer Incidence and Mortality Worldwide: IARC CancerBase No. 11 [Internet]. International Agency for Research on Cancer. http://globocan.iarc.fr, accessed April 4, 2014.

Forman D, Bray F, Brewster DH, et al (Eds). Cancer Incidence in Five Continents, Vol. X (electronic version). Lyon: IARC; 2013. Available from: http://ci5.iarc.fr, accessed November 24, 2013.

International Agency for Research on Cancer. *IARC monographs on the evaluation of the carcinogenic risks to humans: Schistosomes, liver flukes, and Helicobacter pylori.* Vol 61. Lyon: IARC; 1994.

Rastogi T, Hildesheim A, Sinha R. Opportunities for cancer epidemiology in developing countries. *Nat Rev Cancer.* 2004; 4:909-17.

World Health Organization Regional Office for the Eastern Mediterranean. Strategy for cancer prevention and control in the Eastern Mediterranean Region 2009—2013. Geneva: WHO; 2010. Available from: http://applications.emro.who.int/dsaf/EMRPUB_2010_1278.pdf, accessed November 22, 2013.

World Health Organization. Revised global burden of disease (GBD) 2004 Estimates. Geneva: WHO; 2008. Available from: http://www.who.int/healthinfo/global_burden_disease/2004_report_update/en/index.html, accessed November 22, 2013.

Maps and Figures 1 and 2:

Ferlay J, Soerjomataram I, Ervik M, et al. GLOBOCAN 2012 v1.0, Cancer Incidence and Mortality Worldwide: IARC CancerBase No. 11 [Internet]. International Agency for Research on Cancer. http://globocan.iarc.fr, accessed April 4, 2014.

Figure 3:

International Agency for Research on Cancer. Cancer Mortality Database. Lyon; IARC; 2013 [internet]. Available from: http://www-dep.iarc.fr/WHOdb/WHOdb.htm, accessed April 4, 2014.

Cancer Survivorship

Quote:

Mukherjee S. *The Emperor of Maladies: A Biography of Cancer.* New York: Scribner; 2010.

Text, Map, Figures 1 and 2:

Ferlay J, Soerjomataram I, Ervik M, et al. GLOBOCAN 2012 v1.0, Cancer Incidence and Mortality Worldwide: IARC CancerBase No. 11 [Internet]. International Agency for Research on Cancer. http://globocan.iarc.fr, accessed May 19, 2014.

TAKING ACTION

Section Divider

Vineis P, Wild C. Global cancer patterns: Causes and prevention. *Lancet.* 2014; 383(9916):549-57.

The Cancer Continuum

Quote:

Anonymous. Protection of Towns from Fire. February 4, 1735. *The Pennsylvania Gazette.*

Effect of tobacco price increase and reduced consumption:

Jha P. Avoidable global cancer deaths and total deaths from smoking. *Nat Rev Cancer.* 2009;9(9):655-64.

Text:

Brawley O. Avoidable cancer deaths globally. *CA Cancer J Clin.* 2011;61(2):67-8.

Centers for Disease Control and Prevention. *Best practices for comprehensive tobacco control programs- 2007.* Atlanta: U.S. Department of Health and Human Services, Centers for Disease Control and Prevention, National Center for Chronic Disease Prevention and Health Promotion, Office on Smoking and Health; 2007.

International Agency for Research on Cancer. *IARC monographs on the evaluation of carcinogenic risks to humans: Household use of solid fuels and high-temperature frying.* Vol 95. Lyon; IARC; 2010.

Lim SS, Vos T, Flaxman AD, et al. A comparative risk assessment of burden of disease and injury attributable to 67 risk factors and risk factor clusters in 21 regions, 1990-2010: a systematic analysis for the Global Burden of Disease Study 2010. *Lancet.* 2013;380(9859):2224-60.

Lin JS, Eder M, Weinmann S. Behavioral counseling to prevent skin cancer: a systematic review for the U.S. Preventive Services Task Force. *Ann Intern Med.* 2011;154(3):190-201.

Smith RA, Brooks D, Cokkinides V, et al. Cancer screening in the United States, 2013: A review of current American Cancer Society guidelines, current issues in cancer screening, and new guidance on cervical cancer screening and lung cancer screening. *CA Cancer J Clin.* 2013:doi 10.

Thun MJ, DeLancey JO, Center MM, et al. The global burden of cancer: priorities for prevention. *Carcinogenesis.* 2010;31(1):100-110.

World Health Organization. International Programme on Chemical Safety: Air Pollution. 2013. Available from: http://www.who.int/ipcs/assessment/public_health/air_pollution/en/, accessed December 3, 2013.

Figure 1:

Connor SR, Sepulveda Bermedo MC (Eds). *Global Atlas of Palliative Care at the End of Life.* London: Worldwide Palliative Care Alliance; 2014. Available from: http://www.who.int/nmh/Global_Atlas_of_Palliative_Care.pdf, accessed August 14, 2014.

Engholm G FJ, Christensen N, Johannesen TB, et al. NORDCAN: Cancer Incidence, Mortality, Prevalence and Survival in the Nordic Countries, Version 5.2 (December 2012). Available from: http://www.ancr.nu, accessed February 1, 2013.

Ferlay J, Soerjomataram I, Ervik M, et al. GLOBOCAN 2012 v1.0, Cancer Incidence and Mortality Worldwide: IARC CancerBase No. 11 [Internet]. International Agency for Research on Cancer. http://globocan.iarc.fr, accessed December 12, 2013.

Hardcastle JD, Chamberlain JO, Robinson MH, et al. Randomised controlled trial of faecal-occult-blood screening for colorectal cancer. *Lancet.* 1996;348(9040):1472-77.

International Agency for Research on Cancer. *Cancer survival in Africa, Asia, and the Caribbean and Central America.* Lyon; IARC: 2011.

Kronborg O, Fenger C, Olsen J, Jorgensen OD, Sondergaard O. Randomised study of screening for colorectal cancer with faecal-occult-blood test. *Lancet.* 1996;348(9040): 1467-1471.

Lee IM, Shiroma EJ, Lobelo F, et al. Effect of physical inactivity on major non-communicable diseases worldwide: an analysis of burden of disease and life expectancy. *Lancet.* 2012;380(9838):219-29.

Mandel JS, Church TR, Ederer F, Bond JH. Colorectal cancer mortality: effectiveness of biennial screening for fecal occult blood. *J Natl Cancer Inst.* 1999;91(5):434-37.

Sant M, Allemani C, Santaquilani M, et al. EUROCARE-4. Survival of cancer patients diagnosed in 1995-1999. Results and commentary. *Eur J Cancer.* 2009;45(6):931-91.

Figure 2:

Thun MJ, Carter BD, Feskanich D, et al. 50-year trends in smoking-related mortality in the United States. *N Engl J Med.* 2013;368:351-64. Unpublished additional analyses.

Figure 3:

Goldie SJ, O'Shea M, Campos NG, et al. Health and economic outcomes of HPV 16,18 vaccination in 72 GAVI-eligible countries. *Vaccine.* 2008;26(32):4080-93.

Figure 4:

Boschmonar MG, Alvarez YG, García AM, et al. Childhood cancer survival in Cuba. *Eur J Epidemiol.* 2000;16(8):763-7.

Howlader N, Noone AM, Krapcho M, et al (Eds). *SEER Cancer Statistics Review, 1975-2010,* National Cancer Institute. Bethesda, MD, http://seer.cancer.gov/csr/1975_2010/, based on November 2012 SEER data submission, posted to the SEER web site, April 2013.

Myers MH, Heise HW, Li FP, Miller RW. Trends in cancer survival among U.S. white children, 1955-1971. *J Pediatr.* 1975;87(5):815-8.

Perme MP, Jereb B. Trends in survival after childhood cancer in Slovenia between 1957 and 2007. *Pediatr Hematol Oncol.* 2009;26(4):240-51.

Swaminathan R, Rama R, Shanta V. Childhood cancers in Chennai, India, 1990–2001: Incidence and survival. *Int J Cancer.* 2008;122(11):2607-11.

Health Promotion:
A Population and Systems Approach

Quote:

MD Anderson Center. *Division of Cancer Prevention and Population Sciences, MD Anderson Center, Annual Report 2012.* 2012. Available from: http://www.mdanderson.org/education-and-research/departments-programs-and-labs/departments-and-divisions/division-of-cancer-prevention-and-population-sciences/annual-report-fy12-081413.pdf, accessed August 15, 2014.

WHO Global School Health Initiative:

World Health Organization. Global school health initiative. 2013. Available from: http://www.who.int/school_youth_health/gshi/en/, accessed September 3, 2013.

Text:

Linnan L, Bowling M, Childress J, et al. Results of the 2004 National Worksite Health Promotion Survey. *Am J Public Health*. 2008;98:1503-9.

Woolf SH. The power of prevention and what it requires. *JAMA*. 2008;299:2437-9.

World Health Organization. Health Promotion. 2013. Available from: *http://www.who.int/topics/health_promotion/en/*, accessed September 3, 2013.

World Cancer Research Fund / American Institute for Cancer Research. Policy and Action for Cancer Prevention. Food, Nutrition, and Physical Activity: a Global Perspective. Washington, DC: AICR; 2009.

World Health Organization. Global school health initiative. 2013. Available from: *http://www.who.int/school_youth_health/gshi/en/*, accessed September 3, 2013.

Map: Cigarette Warning Labels

World Health Organization. WHO Report on the Global Tobacco Epidemic 2013. Geneva: WHO; 2013. Available from: *http://apps.who.int/iris/bitstream/10665/85380/1/9789241505871_eng.pdf?ua=1*, accessedAugust 15, 2014.

Map: Nutrition Labels

Hawkes C. *Government and voluntary policies on nutrition labelling: a global overview, in Innovations in Food Labelling*. Albert J (Ed). Philadelphia; The Food and Agriculture Organization of the United Nations and Woodhead Publishing; 2010.

Figure 1:

Withall J, Jago R, Fox KR. The effect of a community-based social marketing campaign on recruitment and retention of low-income groups into physical activity programmes. *BMC Public Health*. 2012;12:836.

Figure 2:

World Health Organization. Milestones in Health Promotion: Statements from Global Conferences. Geneva: WHO; 2009.

Tobacco Control

Quote:

Jordans F. *WHO chief slams tobacco firms that 'harass' gov'ts*. 2011. Available from: *http://www.boston.com/lifestyle/health/articles/2011/11/23/who_chief_slams_tobacco_firms_that_harass_govts/*, accessed August 19, 2014.

Plain package labelling in Australia:

Campaign for Tobacco-Free Kids. Tobacco Unfiltered. Available from: *http://www.tobaccofreekids.org/tobacco_unfiltered/tag/plain+packaging*, accessed August 19, 2014.

Text:

Blecher E. *The economics of tobacco control in low- and middle-income countries*. PhD Dissertation. University of Cape Town. 2011.

Campaign for Tobacco-Free Kids. *Cigarette affordability*. 2014. Available from: *http://global.tobaccofreekids.org/files/pdfs/en/TAX_Cigarette_affordability_summary_en.pdf*, accessed March 19, 2014.

Levy DT, Benjakul S, Ross H, Ritthiphakdee B. The role of tobacco control policies in reducing smoking and deaths in a middle income nation: Results from the Thailand SimSmoke simulation model. *Tob Control*. 2008;17(1):53-9.

Levy D, de Almeida LM, Szklo A. The Brazil SimSmoke policy simulation model: The effect of strong tobacco control policies on smoking prevalence and smoking-attributable deaths in a middle income nation. *PLoS Medicine*. 2012;9(11): e1001336.

World Health Organization Framework Convention on Tobacco Control. Parties to the WHO Framework Convention on Tobacco Control. 2014. Available from: *http://www.who.int/fctc/signatories_parties/en/*, accessed March 19, 2014.

World Health Organization. *Tobacco Free Initiative*. 2014. Available from: *http://www.who.int/tobacco/mpower/en/*, accessed March 19, 2014.

Map:

World Health Organization Framework Convention on Tobacco Control. *Parties to the WHO Framework Convention on Tobacco Control*. 2014. Available from: *http://www.who.int/fctc/signatories_parties/en/*, accessed May 1, 2014.

Figure 1:

World Health Organization. *Tobacco Free Initiative*. 2014. Available from: *http://www.who.int/tobacco/mpower/en/*, accessedMarch 19, 2014.

Figure 2:

Levy DT, Benjakul S, Ross H, Ritthiphakdee B. The role of tobacco control policies in reducing smoking and deaths in a middle income model: Results from the Thailand SimSmoke simulation model. *Tob Control*. 2008;17(1):53-9.

Levy D, de Almeida LM, Szklo A. The Brazil SimSmoke policy simulation model: The effect of strong tobacco control policies on smoking prevalence and smoking-attributable deaths in a middle income nation. *PLoS Medicine*. 2012;9(11): e1001336.

Figure 3:

Blecher E. *The economics of tobacco control in low- and middle-income countries*. PhD Dissertation. University of Cape Town. 2011.

Figure 4:

Campaign for Tobacco-Free Kids. *Cigarette Affordability*. 2014. Available from: *http://global.tobaccofreekids.org/files/pdfs/en/TAX_Cigarette_affordability_summary_en.pdf*, accessed March 19, 2014.

Vaccines

Quote:

Desiderius Erasmus Quotes. Available from: *http://www.brainyquote.com/quotes/quotes/d/desiderius148997.html*, accessed August 15, 2014.

Decrease in primary liver cancer in Taiwan:

Chang MH, You SL, Chen CJ, et al. Decreased incidence of hepatocellular carcinoma in hepatitis B vaccinees: a 20-year follow-up study. *J Natl Cancer Inst*. 2009;101(19):1348-55.

Text:

Centers for Disease Control and Prevention. Ten Great Public Health Achievements — Worldwide, 2001–2010. *MMWR Morb Mortal Wkly Rep*. 2011;60:814-18.

Forman D, de Martel C, Lacey CJ, et al. Global burden of human papillomavirus and related diseases. *Vaccine*. 2012;30 Suppl 5:F12-23.

Lozano R, Naghavi M, Foreman K, et al. Global and regional mortality from 235 causes of death for 20 age groups in 1990 and 2010: a systematic analysis for the Global Burden of Disease Study 2010. *Lancet*. 2012;380(9859): 2095-128.

Map: Hepatitis B immunization coverage

World Health Organization. Global Health Observatory Data Repository, Hepatitis B (HepB3) Immunization Coverage of 1-year-olds, Data by Country, 1985-2012 [online database]. Available from: *http://apps.who.int/ghodata/*, accessed August 15, 2014.

Map: Human papillomavirus introduction

World Health Organization. *WHO/Immunization, Vaccines, and Biologicals (IVB) Database*. May 2013. Available from: *http://www.who.int/immunization/en/*, accessed May 29, 2013.

Figure 1:

Forman D, de Martel C, Lacey CJ, et al. Global burden of human papillomavirus and related diseases. *Vaccine*. 2012;30 Suppl 5:F12-23.

Early Detection

Quote:

Buddha Quotes. Available from: *http://www.brainyquote.com/quotes/quotes/b/buddha387356.html*, accessed August 15, 2014.

HPV screening in low- and medium-resource settings could reduce cervical cancer by 30%:

Alliance for Cervical Cancer Prevention. *Preventing cervical cancer worldwide*. Washington, DC: Population Reference Bureau; 2004.

Goldie SJ, Gaffikin L, Goldhaber-Fiebert JD, et al. Cost-effectiveness of cervical cancer screening in 5 developing countries. *N Engl J Med*. 2005;353:2158-68.

Sigmoidoscopy reduces colorectal cancer incidence and mortality:

Atkin WS, Edwards R, Kralj-Hans I, et al. Once-only flexible sigmoidoscopy screening in prevention of colorectal cancer: a multicentre randomised controlled trial. *Lancet*. 2010;375(9726):1624-33.

Text:

Arbyn M, Ronco G, Anttila A, et al. Evidence regarding human papillomavirus testing in secondary prevention of cervical cancer. *Vaccine*. 2012;30 Suppl 5:F88-F99.

Hewitson P, Glasziou P, Watson E, Towler B, Irwig L. Cochrane systematic review of colorectal cancer screening using the fecal occult blood test (hemoccult): an update. *Am J Gastroenterol*. 2008;103(6):1541-9.

Humphrey LL, Deffebach M, Pappas M, et al. Screening for lung cancer with low-dose computed tomography: a systematic review to update the U.S. Preventive Services Task Force recommendation. *Ann Intern Med*. 2013; 159:411-20.

Ilic D, Neuberger MM, Djulbegovic M, Dahm P. Screening for prostate cancer. *Cochrane Database Syst Rev*. 2013;1:CD004720.

International Agency for Research on Cancer. *IARC Handbooks of Cancer Prevention. Volume 7. Breast Cancer Screening*. Lyon: IARC Press; 2007.

International Agency for Research on Cancer. *IARC Handbooks of Cancer Prevention. Volume 10. Cervix Cancer Screening*. Lyon: IARC Press; 2005.

Leung WK, Wu MS, Kakugawa Y, Kim JJ, Yeoh KG, Goh KL, et al. Screening for gastric cancer in Asia: current evidence and practice. *Lancet Oncol*. 2008;9(3):279-87.

Menon U, Griffin M, Gentry-Maharaj A. Ovarian cancer screening--current status, future directions. *Gynecol Oncol*. 2014;132(2):490-5.

Mittra I, Mishra GA, Singh S, et al. A cluster randomized, controlled trial of breast and cervix cancer screening in Mumbai, India: Methodology and interim results after three rounds of screening. *Int J Cancer*. 2010;126(4):976-84.

Ronco G, Dillner J, Elfström KM, et al. Efficacy of HPV-based screening for prevention of invasive cervical cancer: Follow-up of four European randomised controlled trials. *Lancet*. 2014;383(9916):524-32.

Sankaranarayanan R, Esmy PO, Rajkumar R, et al. Effect of visual screening on cervical cancer incidence and mortality in Tamil Nadu, India: A cluster-randomised trial. *Lancet.* 2007;370(9585):398-406.

Sankaranarayanan R, Ramadas K, Thara S, et al. Long term effect of visual screening on oral cancer incidence and mortality in a randomized trial in Kerala, India. *Oral Oncol.* 2013;49(4):314-21.

Sankaranarayanan R, Ramadas K, Thara S, et al. Clinical breast examination: Preliminary results from a cluster randomized controlled trial in India. *J Natl Cancer Inst.* 2011;103(19):1476-80.

Shastri SS, Mittra I, Mishra GA, et al. Effect of VIA Screening by primary health workers: Randomized controlled study in Mumbai, India. *J Natl Cancer Inst.* 2014;106(3):dju009.

Wolff T, Tai E, Miller T. Screening for skin cancer: an update of the evidence for the U.S. Preventive Services Task Force. *Ann Intern Med.* 2009;150(3):194-8.

Maps:
Data provided by the International Agency for Research on Cancer, Section of Early Detection and Prevention, 2014.

Figure 1:
Photos courtesy of the International Agency for Research on Cancer, Section of Early Detection and Prevention, 2014.

Figure 2:
Ferlay J, Bray F, Steliarova-Foucher E, Forman D. Cancer Incidence in Five Continents, CI5plus: IARC CancerBase [Internet]. Lyon, France: International Agency for Research on Cancer; 2014. Available from: http://ci5.iarc.fr, accessed May 23, 2014.

Management and Treatment

Quote:
Farmer P, Frenk J, Knaul FM, et al. Expansion of cancer care and control in countries of low and middle income: a call to action. *Lancet.* 2010;376(9747):1186-93.

Availability of radiotherapy machines:
Abdel-Wahab M, Rosenblatt E, Meghzifene A, et al. Changes in the availability of radiation oncology services in Africa: A report from the International Atomic Energy Agency, 2011. Radiological Society of North America 2011 Scientific Assembly and Annual Meeting, November 26 - December 2, 2011, Chicago IL.

Barton MB, Frommer M, Shafiq J. Role of radiotherapy in cancer control in low-income and middle-income countries. *Lancet Oncol.* 2006;7:584-95.

Ekortari A, Ndom P, Sacks A. A study of patients who appear with far advanced cancer at Yaounde General Hospital, Cameroon, Africa. *Psychooncology.* 2007;16(3):255-57.

Gomes Junior SC, Almeida RT. Simulation model for estimating the cancer care infrastructure required by the public health system. *Pan Am J Public Health.* 2009;25(2):113-9.

The Swedish Council on Technology Assessment in Health Care. Radiotherapy for cancer – a systematic literature review. *Acta Oncol.* 1996;2:35.

Van de Werf E, Verstraete J, Lievens Y. The cost of radiotherapy in a decade of technology evolution. *Radiother Oncol.* 2012;102:148-53.

Williams MV, Drinkwater KL. Geographical variation in radiotherapy services across the UK in 2007 and the effect of deprivation, *Clin Oncol.* 2009;21:431-40.

Text:
Abdel-Wahab M, Rosenblatt E, Meghzifene A, et al. *Changes in the availability of radiation oncology services in Africa:*

A report from the International Atomic Energy Agency, 2011. Radiological Society of North America 2011 Scientific Assembly and Annual Meeting, November 26 – December 2, 2011, Chicago IL.

Adesina A, Chumba D, Nelson AM, et al. Improvement of pathology in sub-Saharan Africa. *Lancet Oncol.* 2013;14(4):e152-7.

Barton MB, Frommer M, Shafiq J. Role of radiotherapy in cancer control in low-income and middle-income countries. *Lancet Oncol.* 2006;7:584-95.

Boyle P, D'Onofrio A, Maisonneuve P, et al. Measuring progress against cancer in Europe: has the 15% decline targeted for 2000 come about? *Ann Oncol.* 2003;14: 1312-25.

Coleman MP, Quaresma M, Berrino F, et al., for the CONCORD Working Group. Cancer survival in five continents: a worldwide population-based study (CONCORD). *Lancet Oncol.* 2008;9:730–56.

Elzawawy A. Science and affordability of cancer drugs and radiotherapy in the world— Win-win scenarios. In: Mohan R, editors. *Advances in Cancer Management.* Rijeka: InTech; 2012. p.255-278. Available from: *http://www.intechopen.com/articles/show/title/science-and-affordability-of-cancer-drugs-and-radiotherapy-in-the-world*, accessed July 11, 2014.

Ferlay J, Soerjomataram I, Ervik M, et al. GLOBOCAN 2012 v1.0, Cancer Incidence and Mortality Worldwide: IARC CancerBase No. 11 [Internet]. Lyon, France: International Agency for Research on Cancer; 2013. Available from: http://globocan.iarc.fr, accessed December 12, 2013.

Hanna TP, Kangolle ACT. Cancer control in developing countries: Using health data and health services research to measure and improve access, quality and efficiency. *BMC International Health Hum Rights.* 2010;10:24.

Kingham TP, Alatise OI, Vanderpuye V, et al. Treatment of cancer in sub-Saharan Africa. *Lancet Oncol.* 2013;14(4):e158-67.

Ott JJ, Ullrich A, Miller AB. The importance of early symptom recognition in the context of early detection and cancer survival. *Eur J Cancer.* 2009;45:2743–48.

Patel JD, Galsky MD, Chagpar AB, Pyle D, Loehrer PJ Sr. Role of American Society of Clinical Oncology in low- and middle-income countries. *J Clin Oncol.* 2011;29(22):3097-102.

Price P, Sikora K. *Treatment of cancer,* 5th ed. London: Arnold Hodder, 2008.

Sener SF, Grey N. The global burden of cancer. *J Surgical Oncol.* 2005;92: 1–3.

Sullivan R, Peppercorn J, Sikora K, et al. Delivering affordable cancer care in high income countries. *Lancet Oncol.* 2011;12: 933-80.

Van de Werf E, Verstraete J, Lievens Y. The cost of radiotherapy in a decade of technology evolution. *Radiother Oncol.* 2012;102:148-53.

Map: Radiotherapy coverage
Data provided by the International Atomic Energy Agency (IAEA), 2014.

Methods: For this estimation, the assumptions are that 60% of cancer patients need radiotherapy, and one radiotherapy machine can treat 500 new patients per year (based on references below). Data on cancer incidence generated from GLOBOCAN 2012 (IARC). Radiotherapy machines are self-reported by countries on a voluntary basis to the IAEA's Directory of Radiotherapy Centres (DIRAC). Information on countries with no radiotherapy machines was provided by IAEA's Programme of Action for Cancer Therapy (PACT) (Dec 2013).

References for radiotherapy map:

Boyle P, D'Onofrio A, Maisonneuve P, et al. Measuring progress against cancer in Europe: has the 15% decline targeted for 2000 come about? *Annals Oncol.* 2003;14:1312-25.

Ferlay J, Soerjomataram I, Ervik M, et al. GLOBOCAN 2012 v1.0, Cancer Incidence and Mortality Worldwide: IARC CancerBase No. 11 [Internet]. Lyon, France: International Agency for Research on Cancer; 2013. Available from: http://globocan.iarc.fr, accessed December 12, 2013.

Ringborg U, Bergqvist D, Brorsson B, et al. The Swedish council on technology assessment in health care (SBU) systematic overview of radiotherapy for cancer. *Acta Oncol.* 2003;42:357–65.

Van de Werf E, Verstraete J, Lievens Y. The cost of radiotherapy in a decade of technology evolution. *Radiother Oncol.* 2012;102:148-53.

Figure 1:
World Health Organization. Essential drugs for cancer chemotherapy: Memorandum from a WHO meeting. *Bull WHO.* 1985;63: 999-1002.

World Health Organization. *WHO Model List of Essential Medicines, 18th List.* April 2013. Available from: *http://www.who.int/medicines/publications/essentialmedicines/18th_EML_Final_web_8Jul13.pdf*, accessed July 11, 2014.

Figure 2:
International Atomic Energy Agency. Available from: *http://cancer.iaea.org/agart.asp*, accessed July 11, 2014.

Figure 3:
Adesina A, Chumba D, Nelson AM, et al. Improvement of pathology in sub-Saharan Africa. *Lancet Oncol.* 2013;14(4):e152-7.

Pain Control

Quote:
Life Before Death. Dir. Mike Hill. DVD. Melbourne: Moonshine Movies; 2012.

More than 2.7 million people die in pain each year:
Treat the Pain. *Access to essential pain medicines brief (2011 data).* 2013. Available from: *http://www.treatthepain.org/*, accessed January 7, 2014.

Text:
Foley KM, Wagner JL, Joranson DE, Gelband H. Pain control for people with cancer and AIDS. In: *Disease Control Priorities in Developing Countries.* 2nd ed. New York: Oxford University Press; 2006. p. 981–94.

Treat the Pain. *Data.* 2013. Available from: *http://www.treatthepain.org/*, accessed January 7, 2014.

World Health Organization. WHO Model Lists of Essential Medicines. 2013. Available from: *http://www.who.int/medicines/publications/essentialmedicines/en/*, accessed August 15, 2014.

Map:
Treat the Pain. *Access to essential pain medicines brief (2011 data).* 2013. Available from: *http://www.treatthepain.org/*, accessed January 7, 2014

Cancer Registries

Quote:
Global Initiative for Cancer Registry Development. *Let's face the facts.* Lyon, France: International Agency for Research on Cancer. 2012. Available at: *http://gicr.iarc.fr/files/resources/20120822-BrochureGICR_en.pdf.* Accessed July 11, 2014.

Only 9 low- and medium HDI countries have high-quality registry data:
Global Initiative for Cancer Registry Development. *Let's face the facts.* Lyon, France: International Agency for Research on Cancer. 2014. Available at: *http://gicr.iarc.fr/files/resources/20140424-Brochure2014.pdf.* Accessed July 11, 2014.

Text:
Bray F, Znaor A, Cueva P, et al. The role and status of population-based cancer registration. In: *Planning and developing population-based cancer registration in low- and middle-income settings.* IARC Technical Report No. 23. Lyon; IARC. pp. 3-7.

Doll R, Payne P, Waterhouse JAH (Eds). *Cancer Incidence in Five Continents, Vol. I.* Geneva; Union Internationale Contre le Cancer; 1966.

Forman D, Bray F, Brewster DH, et al (Eds). *Cancer Incidence in Five Continents, Vol. X* (electronic version) Lyon: IARC; 2013. Available from: *http://ci5.iarc.fr/CI5-X,* accessed July 11, 2014.

Mathers CD, Fat DM, Inoue M, Rao C, Lopez AD. Counting the dead and what they died from: an assessment of the global status of cause of death data. *Bull World Health Organ.* 2005;83(3):171-7.

Map: Quality of cancer registry data:
Bray F, Znaor A, Cueva P, et al. The role and status of population-based cancer registration. In: *Planning and Developing Population-Based Cancer Registration in Low- and Middle-Income Settings.* IARC Technical Report No. 23. Lyon; IARC. pp. 3-7.

Map: Quality of vital registration data:
Ferlay J, Soerjomataram I, Ervik M, et al. GLOBOCAN 2012 v1.0, Cancer Incidence and Mortality Worldwide: IARC CancerBase No. 11 [Internet]. Lyon, France: International Agency for Research on Cancer; 2013. Available from: *http://globocan.iarc.fr,* accessed July 11, 2014.

Mathers CD, Fat DM, Inoue M, Rao C, Lopez AD. Counting the dead and what they died from: an assessment of the global status of cause of death data. *Bull World Health Organ.* 2005;83(3):171-7.

Figure 1:
Curado MP, Edwards B, Shin HR, et al. (Eds). *Cancer Incidence in Five Continents, Vol. IX.* IARC Scientific Publications, No. 160. Lyon: IARC; 2007.

Doll R, Muir CS, Waterhouse JAH (Eds). *Cancer Incidence in Five Continents, Vol. II.* Geneva; Union Internationale Contre le Cancer; 1970.

Doll R, Payne P, Waterhouse JAH (Eds). *Cancer Incidence in Five Continents, Vol. I.* Geneva; Union Internationale Contre le Cancer; 1966.

Forman D, Bray F, Brewster DH, et al (Eds). *Cancer Incidence in Five Continents, Vol. X* (electronic version) Lyon: IARC; 2013. Available from: *http://ci5.iarc.fr/CI5-X,* accessed July 11, 2014.

Muir CS, Waterhouse J, Mack T, et al (Eds). *Cancer Incidence in Five Continents, Vol. V.* IARC Scientific Publications, No. 88. Lyon: IARC; 1987.

Parkin, DM, Muir CS, Whelan SL, et al (Eds). *Cancer Incidence in Five Continents, Vol. VI.* IARC Scientific Publications,

Parkin, DM, Whelan SL, Ferlay J, et al (Eds). *Cancer Incidence in Five Continents, Vol. VIII.* IARC Scientific Publications, No. 155. Lyon: IARC; 2002.

Parkin, DM, Whelan SL, Ferlay J, et al (Eds). *Cancer Incidence in Five Continents, Vol. VII.* IARC Scientific Publications, No. 143. Lyon: IARC; 1997.

Waterhouse J, Muir CS, Correa P, Powell J (Eds). *Cancer Incidence in Five Continents, Vol. III.* IARC Scientific Publications, No. 15. Lyon: IARC; 1976.

Waterhouse J, Muir CS, Shanmugaratnam K, Powell J (Eds). *Cancer Incidence in Five Continents, Vol. IV.* IARC Scientific Publications, No. 42. Lyon: IARC; 1982.

Figure 2:
Forman D, Bray F, Brewster DH, et al (Eds). *Cancer Incidence in Five Continents, Vol. X* (electronic version) Lyon: IARC; 2013. Available from: *http://ci5.iarc.fr/CI5-X,* accessed July 11, 2014.

Mathers CD, Fat DM, Inoue M, Rao C, Lopez AD. Counting the dead and what they died from: an assessment of the global status of cause of death data. *Bull World Health Organ.* 2005;83(3):171-7.

Research

Quote:
Gaither CC, Cavazos-Gaither AE (Eds). *Scientifically speaking: A book of quotations,* 2nd Ed. London: The Institute of Physics; 2000. p. 333.

Medicines and fundamental biology dominate:
Eckhouse S, Lewison G, Sullivan R. Trends in the global funding and activity of cancer research. *Mol Oncol.* 2008;2(1):20-32.

9% of cancer research is surgical:
Purushotham AD, Lewison G, Sullivan R. The state of research and development in global cancer surgery. *Ann Surg.* 2012;255(3):427-32.

Text:
Cazap E. A vision of independent clinical research in South America. *ASCO Post.* 2014;5(8).

Eckhouse S, Lewison G, Sullivan R. Trends in the global funding and activity of cancer research. *Mol Oncol.* 2008;2(1):20-32.

Seruga B, Sadikov A, Cazap EL, et al. Barriers and challenges to global clinical cancer research. *Oncologist.* 2014;19(1):61-7.

Shastri SS, Mittra I, Mishra GA, et al. Effect of VIA screening by primary health workers: randomized controlled study in Mumbai, India. *J Natl Cancer Inst.* 2014;106(3):dju009.

Strother RM, Asirwa FC, Busakhala NB, et al. AMPATH-Oncology: A model for comprehensive cancer care in sub-Saharan Africa. *J Cancer Policy.* 2013;1(3):e42-e8.

Sullivan R. Policy challenges for cancer research: a call to arms. *eCancerMedicalScience.* 2007;1(53).

Sullivan R, Eckhouse S, Lewison G. Using bibliometrics to inform cancer research policy and spending. In: *Monitoring financial flows for health research 2007.* Geneva: Global Forum for Health Research; 2008. p. 67-78.

Sullivan R, Kowalczyk JR, Agarwal B, et al. New policies to address the global burden of childhood cancers. *Lancet Oncol.* 2013;14(3):e125-35.

Sullivan R, Purushotham A. Towards an international cancer control plan: Policy solutions for the global cancer epidemic. International Centre for Migration, Health and Development, 2010.

Inset: Partnerships in India
Sullivan R, Badwe RA, Rath GK, et al. Cancer research in India: National priorities, global results. *Lancet Oncol.* 2014;15(6):e213-22.

Figures 1 and 4:
Data provided by the Institute of Cancer Policy, UK, 2014.

Figure 2:
Eckhouse S, Sullivan R. A survey of public funding of cancer research in the European union. *PLoS Med.* 2006;3(7):e267.

Figure 3:
Purushotham AD, Lewison G, Sullivan R. The state of research and development in global cancer surgery. *Ann Surg.* 2012;255(3):427-32.

Investing in Cancer Prevention

Quote:
Mahatma Gandhi Quotes. Available from: *http://www.brainyquote.com/quotes/quotes/m/mahatmagan109078.html,* accessed August 15, 2014.

HPV vaccine cost-effectiveness:
Goldie SJ, O'Shea M, Campos NG, Diaz M, Sweet S, Kim S-Y. Health and economic outcomes of HPV 16, 18 vaccination in 72 GAVI-eligible countries. *Vaccine.* 2008;26(32):4080-93.

Text:
Elkin EB, Bach PB. Cancer's next frontier: Addressing high and increasing costs. *JAMA.* 2010;303(11):1086-7.

Goldie SJ, Gaffikin L, Goldhaber-Fiebert JD, et al. Cost-Effectiveness of Cervical-Cancer Screening in Five Developing Countries. *N Engl J Med.* 2005;353(20):2158-68.

Laxminarayan R, Chow J, Shahid-Salles SA. Intervention cost-effectiveness: Overview of main messages. In: Jamison DT, Breman JG, Measham AR, et al., eds. *Disease control priorities in developing countries.* Washington (DC): World Bank; 2006. p. 35-86.

National Heart Lung and Blood Institute. *NHLBI Fact Book, Fiscal Year 2012.* Bethesda, MD: NHLBI; 2012.

World Health Organization. *Scaling up action against noncommunicable diseases: How much will it cost?* Geneva: WHO; 2011.

Figure 1:
Australian Government. *Budget at a Glance.* Available from: *http://www.budget.gov.au/2013-14/content/at_a_glance/html/at_a_glance.htm,* accessed April 30, 2014.

Chen P-C, Lee Y-C, Tsai S-T, Lai C-K. A cost-benefit analysis of the outpatient smoking cessation services in Taiwan from a societal viewpoint. *Nicotine Tob Res.* 2012;14(5):522-30.

Directorate-General of Budget, Accounting and Statistics of Taiwan. *Central Government General Budget.* Available from: *http://eng.dgbas.gov.tw/ct.asp?xItem=33683&CtNode=6002&mp=2,* accessed April 30, 2014.

Hurley SF, Matthews JP. Cost-effectiveness of the Australian national tobacco campaign. *Tob Control.* 2008;17(6):379-84.

Government of the Netherlands. *Expenditure in 2014.* Available from: *http://www.government.nl/issues/budget/revenue-and-expenditure-in-2014/expenditure-in-2014,* accessed April 30, 2014.

Lammers M, Kok L. Cost benefit analysis of dietary treatment. Dutch Society of Dietitians; 2012. Available from: *http://www.seo.nl/uploads/media/2012-76a_Cost-benefit_analysis_of_dietary_treatment.pdf,* accessed April 30, 2014.

National Colorectal Cancer Roundtable. *Increasing colorectal cancer screening – saving lives and saving dollars: Screening 50 to 84 year olds reduces cancer costs to Medicare.* [Internet]. 2007 Sep. Available from: *http://action.acscan.org/site/DocServer/Increasing_Colorectal_Cancer_Screening_-_Saving_Lives_an.pdf?docID=18927,* accessed April 30, 2014.

National School Lunch Program. *NSLP Fact Sheet*. 2013. Available from: *http://www.fns.usda.gov/sites/default/files/NSLPFactSheet.pdf*, accessed September 1, 2013.

Figure 2:
European Commission. *EU budget 2009 - Financial Report*. 2010. Available from: *http://ec.europa.eu/budget/library/biblio/publications/2009/fin_report/fin_report_09_en.pdf*, accessed April 30, 2014.

Luengo-Fernandez R, Leal J, Gray A, Sullivan R. Economic burden of cancer across the European Union: a population-based cost analysis. *Lancet Oncol*. 2013;14(12):1165-74.

Figure 3:
World Health Organization. *Scaling up action against noncommunicable diseases: How much will it cost?* Geneva: WHO; 2011.

METHODS:
Ten countries with the largest estimated age-world-standardized cervical cancer mortality rate in 2012 according to GLOBOCAN. Estimates include the cost of one-off screening among women aged 35 to 45 years using visual inspection with acetic acid (VIA), and immediate treatment of precancerous lesions using cryotherapy for those women who screen positive. The estimates reflect per-capita annual average cost of scaling up prevention of cervical cancer over the period 2010-2025 and are calculated based on the NCD costing tool developed by the World Health Organization. The target coverage level was set at 80% for 2025.

Figure 4:
Goldie SJ, O'Shea M, Campos NG, Diaz M, Sweet S, Kim S-Y. Health and economic outcomes of HPV 16, 18 vaccination in 72 GAVI-eligible countries. *Vaccine*. 2008;26(32):4080-93.

METHODS:
Assumes vaccination of 70% of a single birth cohort of 9-year-old girls in 2007 at cost of 25 international dollars (approximately US$5 per dose) per vaccinated girl.

Leveraging Existing Infrastructure

Quote:
Farmer P, Frenk J, Knaul FM, et al. Expansion of cancer care and control in countries of low and middle income: A call to action. *Lancet*. 2010;376(9747):1186-93.

Text:
Centers for Disease Control and Prevention. Global Health – Health Protection. Field Epidemiology Training Program (FETP). Available from: *http://www.cdc.gov/globalhealth/fetp/*, accessed July 11, 2014.

Farmer P, Frenk J, Knaul FM, et al. Expansion of cancer care and control in countries of low and middle income: a call to action. *Lancet*. 2010;376(9747):1186-93.

Pink Ribbon Red Ribbon. Available from: *http://pinkribbonredribbon.org/*, accessed July 11, 2014.

Map:
Data provided by the Centers for Disease Control and Prevention, Field Epidemiology Training Program, 2014, and Pink Ribbon Red Ribbon, 2014.

Figure 1:
Centers for Disease Control and Prevention. *Global Health – Health Protection. Field Epidemiology Training Program (FETP)*. Available from: *http://www.cdc.gov/globalhealth/fetp/*, accessed July 11, 2014.

Photo courtesy of the CDC Field Epidemiology Training Program, 2014.

Figure 2:
Data provided by Pink Ribbon Red Ribbon, 2014.
Photo courtesy of Pink Ribbon Red Ribbon, 2014.

Figure 3:
Global Alliance for Vaccines and Immunisation (GAVI). Available from: *http://www.gavialliance.org/*, accessed July 11, 2014.

Farmer P, Frenk J, Knaul FM, et al. Expansion of cancer care and control in countries of low and middle income: a call to action. *Lancet*. 2010;376(9747):1186-93.

Photo courtesy of Pink Ribbon Red Ribbon, 2014.

Uniting Organizations

Quote:
Union for International Cancer Control. *Annual Report – 2013*. 2013. Available from: *http://www.uicc.org/2013-annual-report*, accessed August 18, 2014.

Text:
Union for International Cancer Control. *World Cancer Declaration 2013*. 2013. Available from: *http://www.uicc.org/world-cancer-declaration*, accessed July 11, 2014.

Map:
Data provided by the Union for International Cancer Control, 2014.

Figure 1:
Union for International Cancer Control. *Convening*. Available from: *http://www.uicc.org/convening*, accessed July 11, 2014.

Figure 2:
Union for International Cancer Control. *World Cancer Declaration 2013*. 2013. Available from: *http://www.uicc.org/world-cancer-declaration*, accessed July 11, 2014.

Global Relay For Life:

Text:
American Cancer Society. *Global Relay for Life*. 2014. Available from: *http://www.relayforlife.org/learn/relayeventsforeveryone/international-relay-for-life*, accessed August 15, 2014.

American Cancer Society. *Global Relay for Life 2012*. 2012. Available from: *http://www.youtube.com/watch?v=Xe5AunMcdBI*, accessed August 19, 2014.

Map and Figures 1 and 2:
Data provided by Global Relay For Life, American Cancer Society, 2014.

Photos:
Photos courtesy of Global Relay For Life, American Cancer Society, 2014.

Policies and Legislation:

Quote:
Ki-Moon B. *Remarks to General Assembly meeting on the Prevention and Control of Non-Communicable Diseases. UN News Centre*. 2011. Available from: *http://www.un.org/apps/news/infocus/sgspeeches/search_full.asp?statID=1299*, accessed August 15, 2014.

Economic toll of NCDs in low- and middle- income countries to reach US$21 trillion:
The NCD Alliance. *NCD Alliance Briefing Paper: Tackling non-communicable diseases to enhance sustainable development*. 2014. Available from: *http://ncdalliance.org/sites/default/files/NCD%20Alliance%20-%20NCDs%20and%20Sustainable%20Development%20Brief_0.pdf*, accessed August 15, 2014.

Text:
Campaign for Tobacco Free Kids. 2014. Available from: *http://global.tobaccofreekids.org/en*, accessed August 15, 2014.

Global Alliance for Vaccines and Immunisation (GAVI). *Human papillomavirus vaccine support*. Available from: *http://www.gavialliance.org/support/nvs/human-papillomavirus-vaccine-support/*, accessed August 15, 2014.

World Health Organization. *Global Health Observatory data repository, hepatitis b (hepb3) immunization coverage of 1-year-olds, data by country, 1985-2012 [online database]*. Available from: *http://apps.who.int/ghodata/*, accessed August 15, 2014.

World Health Organization. *WHO global action plan 2013-2020 for the prevention and control of noncommunicable diseases*. 2013. Available from: *http://apps.who.int/iris/bitstream/10665/94384/1/9789241506236_eng.pdf?ua=1*, accessed August 15, 2014.

World Health Organization. *WHO 2013 non-communicable disease country capacity survey* (unpublished results). Geneva: World Health Organization; 2014.

Map:
World Health Organization. *WHO 2013 non-communicable disease country capacity survey (unpublished results)*. Data provided by the Department of Prevention of Non-communicable Diseases, Non-communicable Diseases and Mental Cluster, World Health Organization, 2014.

METHODS:
The survey included 178 WHO member states. A member state was considered to have an operational cancer control policy if the country indicated that it has either a national non-communicable disease control policy that includes cancer or a national standalone cancer control policy, or both. A member state was considered not to have an operational cancer control policy if it did not indicate it has a cancer control policy. Countries with missing data were not survey recipients.

Figure 1:
Bloom DE, Cafiero ET, Jané-Llopis E, et al. *The global economic burden of noncommunicable diseases*. Geneva: World Economic Forum; 2011.

The NCD Alliance. *NCD Alliance Briefing Paper: Tackling non-communicable diseases to enhance sustainable development*. 2014. Available from: *http://ncdalliance.org/sites/default/files/NCD%20Alliance%20-%20NCDs%20and%20Sustainable%20Development%20Brief_0.pdf*, accessed August 15, 2014.

Figure 2:
World Health Organization. WHO global action plan 2013-2020 for the prevention and control of noncommunicable diseases. 2013. Available from: *http://apps.who.int/iris/bitstream/10665/94384/1/9789241506236_eng.pdf?ua=1*, accessed August 15, 2014.

SOURCES AND METHODS

APPENDICES

Risk Factors for Cancer

Population: United Nations, Department of Economic and Social Affairs. UN World Population Prospects, 2012 revision. Available from: *http://esa.un.org/unpd/wpp/Excel-Data/population.htm*, accessed April 1, 2014.

Smoking prevalence, youths (10-14 years) and adults (15 years and older): Data provided by the Institute for Health Metrics and Evaluation, 2014.

Prevalence of overweight and obese: World Health Organization. Global Health Observatory Data Repository, Overweight (Body Mass Index > 25) Data by Country, 2008 [online database]. Available from: *http://apps.who.int/ghodata/*, accessed November 9, 2012.

Hepatitis B immunization coverage of one-year-olds: World Health Organization. Global Health Observatory Data Repository, Hepatitis B (HepB3) Immunization Coverage of 1-year-olds, Data by Country, 1985-2012 [online database]. Available from: *http://apps.who.int/ghodata/*, accessed August 15, 2014.

Risk of getting cancer: Ferlay J, Soerjomataram I, Ervik M, et al. GLOBOCAN 2012 v1.0, Cancer Incidence and Mortality Worldwide: IARC CancerBase No. 11 [Internet]. Available from: *http://globocan.iarc.fr*, accessed December 12, 2013.

Statistics on Cancer

Ferlay J, Soerjomataram I, Ervik M, et al. GLOBOCAN 2012 v1.0, Cancer Incidence and Mortality Worldwide: IARC CancerBase No. 11 [Internet]. Available from: *http://globocan.iarc.fr*, accessed December 12, 2013.

History of Cancer

Mackay J, Jemal A, Lee NC, Parkin DM. *The Cancer Atlas*. First Ed. Atlanta: American Cancer Society; 2006.

Aberle DR, Adams AM, Berg CD, et al. Reduced lung-cancer mortality with low-dose computed tomographic screening. *N Engl J Med.* 2011;365:395-409.

US Food and Drug Administration. *FDA Licenses New Vaccine for Prevention of Cervical Cancer and Other Diseases in Females Caused by Human Papillomavirus: Rapid Approval Marks Major Advancement in Public Health.* Available from: *http://www.fda.gov/NewsEvents/Newsroom/PressAnnouncements/2006/ucm108666.htm*, accessed August 19, 2014.

Photos:

American Cancer Society courtesy of the American Cancer Society.

E. Cuyler Hammond and Daniel Horn courtesy of the American Cancer Society.

Dr. Min Chiu Li courtesty of the National Cancer Institute.

Mammography image courtesy of the American Cancer Society.

Glossary

Ferlay J, Bray F, Steliarova-Foucher E, Forman D. Cancer Incidence in Five Continents, CI5*plus*: IARC CancerBase [Internet]. Lyon, France: International Agency for Research on Cancer; 2014. Available from: http://ci5.iarc.fr, accessed May 23, 2014.

Ferlay J, Soerjomataram I, Ervik M, et al. GLOBOCAN 2012 v1.0, Cancer Incidence and Mortality Worldwide: IARC CancerBase No. 11 [Internet]. Available from: *http://globocan.iarc.fr*, accessed December 12, 2013.

Mackay J, Jemal A, Lee NC, Parkin DM. *The Cancer Atlas*. First Ed. Atlanta: American Cancer Society; 2006.

National Cancer Institute (US). *NCI Dictionary of Cancer Terms*. Available from: *http://www.cancer.gov/dictionary*, accessed July 1, 2014.

INDEX